Amazing Grace

Autobiography of a Survivor

Grace Halloran, Ph.D

An angry young woman, in Federal prison at eighteen; later, told she's going blind from a genetic disorder; as a mother, shocked to hear that her infant son is also destined to go blind. Stirred to action, she does what the medical world says is impossible...

"It was a distinct pleasure for me to be asked to review *Amazing Grace: Autobiography of a Survivor*. Although I first met Grace Halloran several years ago, reading her story gave me an even greater appreciation for this remarkable woman.

She survived youthful mistakes and indiscretions by accepting responsibility, enduring the consequences, and anchoring herself in a bedrock faith that her life was destined to get better. Devastated by her separation from her first child, she never gave up hope for a future reunion.

Confronted with a diagnosis of retinitis pigmentosa and a sentence of certain blindness, she rejected the verdict of established medicine and set about to find treatment for this untreatable condition. At first, she had hoped only to find help for herself and her young son, who was also at risk for the disease. Along the way, she helped countless others – myself included.

All memorable biographies embody a struggle of the human spirit. *Amazing Grace* is no exception. Against pain, tragedy, and darkness, her extraordinary spirit struggled and prevailed. Her life is a vivid testament to the old adage that the only difference between stumbling blocks and stepping stones is how we use them.

Through it all, Grace Halloran has not merely survived, she has triumphed!"

Willie L. Brown, Jr.
Former Speaker of the California Assembly

"Hers is a journey of strength through extraordinary adversity. She applies the wisdom gained from her experience to provide remarkable insight, while instilling courage, faith, and joy. She brings the message that we can indeed heal ourselves, our lives, and relationships, while creating miracles along the way."

Bruce L. Erickson
International Consultant on Issues of Global Change

"*Amazing Grace* is an inspiring, provocative book that shows how grit and determination can lead to triumph over serious personal problems. Grace's story is an exciting testament to the human spirit."

Jeffery Hewson
QVC Network

"*Amazing Grace* will inspire thousands to show their children that early mistakes can be overcome, that a successful life is possible."

Loren Dunton
President, National Center for Financial Education Author of Prime Time: How to Enjoy the Best Years of Your Life

AMAZING GRACE

Amazing Grace

Autobiography of a Survivor

Grace Halloran, Ph.D

Second Edition
With a new Introduction and
an Afterword by
Damon P. Miller II, MD, CNP

Library of Congress Control Number: 2017914776
ISBN: 978-1-946036-16-2

First edition published 1993

Cover Design: Carlyle Coash
Second edition published 2017
10 9 8 7 6 5 4 3 2 1
OrganicMD Media
PO Box 50399
Palo Alto, CA 94303

ACKNOWLEDGEMENTS for the First Edition

ACKNOWLEDGEMENTS for the First Edition

Special thanks to all the people who have supported me, particularly my niece Amber, who made me feel like a real writer. I am also grateful to George Trim, my publisher, who saw my potential; to Tamsen George and Mary Erpelding for their editorial support; and to my final editor John Niendorff, who went far beyond the call of duty in helping me finish this book.

DEDICATION

To my mother, for bringing me into the world, and to my children for teaching me what love is all about.

Introduction to Amazing Grace: Autobiography of a Survivor

You are about to read the story of an amazing woman. When I first met Grace Halloran, Ph.D., in 1997, she was presenting the results of a rather impressive research study she had conducted with the help of a San Francisco ophthalmologist to a medical conference in Minnesota. This Minnesota stop just one of many, as her findings had garnered invitations from prestigious conferences around the world.

Her research centered on a program to treat degenerative eye disease. I had been taught in medical school that all of the degenerative retinopathy's (diseases affecting the retina) were untreatable—they did not spontaneously improve, only progressively worsened. Yet here was Grace, not a physician, presenting data that showed marked improvement of vision in people with these "untreatable" diseases. Two other optometrists who had implemented Grace's program presented in Minnesota, and their data revealed the same success.

Grace's autobiography does not begin with Grace the Ph.D. and medical researcher. Instead, Grace takes us to a less flattering place, when she was a young woman a bit adrift in her life, exercising more than her share of bad judgment. Why show us Grace the troubled young woman? Because her early struggles forged the courage that she would later need to overcome the vicious eye disease that afflicted herself and her son, as well as a hostile medical establishment.

As we follow Grace along her journey overcoming retinitis pigmentosa, we can see that Grace's journey is a hero's journey. If Grace were alive, she would slap me for using this kind of praise to describe her life; but it's a proper description. Though, perhaps it's truer, and stronger praise, to say Grace's journey is a mother's journey.

The birth of Grace's son is perhaps the pivotal moment in her story. Her son's doctors diagnosed him with retinitis pigmentosa when he was only months old, and warned that he would be all but blind by the time he was in high school. Grace had long tolerated this sort of hopelessness from doctors when they would talk to her about her own disease, but refused to accept it when it concerned her son.

From her college studies, she knew that the body has an incredible ability to heal itself. It seemed wrong that the body could not heal the eyes, just as it could every other part of itself. Eventually, she told her son's doctors that they themselves were hopeless and suffering from some serious deficiencies of imagination.

Fortunately, Grace lived in Northern California, home to some of the most radical imaginations when it comes to healing. With the help of several gifted physicians, Grace pioneered a program that preserved her son's vision, restored her own vision and benefited the vision of everyone in her family that was willing to work with her in the Visual Healing Program. Its development was by no means a smooth road, but its bumps and pitfalls reveal a great deal about modern medicine and our body's capacity for healing.

Grace's work has become a focus in my practice, yet when I attended that conference in Minnesota in the dead of winter, I had no idea I would meet Grace, and really wasn't focused on degenerative eye diseases at all, despite it afflicting many of my patients. It turned out Grace lived barely 20 miles from me in California, and it did not take long for us to start working together to restore eyesight to people who were supposed to go blind.

I am honored to have known and worked with Grace Halloran Ph.D, and to continue her work today.

Damon P. Miller II, MD, CNP

BetterEyeHealth.com

OrganicMD.com

MicrocurrentStimulation.com

Contents

1

NO SUCH THING
AS A FREE DRINK

When I was a little girl, I always dreamed of being the "first". The first woman jet pilot or perhaps the first woman on the moon. I never dreamed I'd be the first eighteen-year-old girl that a certain Federal judge would send to prison. That wasn't a dream of mine at all.

Stealing the old Chevrolet was not premeditated. Rather, it was an impulsive statement about how my life was going. I had been living with my lover, a handsome, sexy, unmotivated man. Neither of us had jobs. All the dancing and drinking at the clubs downtown was not filling up the unhappy space inside of me.

The criminal act itself was a fluke. It started when I was sitting in a bar, pretending to be someone else—someone older, someone smiling, talking to the men on either side. I lied to the bartender, telling him it was my birthday. Usually the bartender bought the first drink on the house, and the guys in the bar continued the free flow of booze if they thought they could get somewhere with me. It was a game I learned a while back to get free drinks.

The middle-aged man sitting on my right had class. He bought a bottle of the house champagne. That impressed me, and from then on, my attention focused on him. When he suggested that we take a ride, I was in a good mood and had drunk more than my share of free drinks.

My boyfriend Jack was home pouting. We had argued earlier in the day. We were too young and very spoiled. Neither of us liked to lose an argument. He stayed home to punish me, and I went out to hurt him. In that impulsive act, I was the one who would end up paying for a long time.

Leaving the bar with a stranger was another way to get back at Jack. He deserved it, I told myself, justifying my reckless, dangerous behavior.

When my "date" drove into the cheap motel in the more sleazy section of South San Francisco, I didn't say anything. Something inside me started to come unglued, but I couldn't quite put my finger on it.

Why do all men want sex? I didn't really know or like this guy, yet here we were, checking into a drive-in motel. A cheap date could probably rent rooms here by the hour. My stomach was beginning to get tight, and I was sobering up fast.

I was also getting angry, waiting in the car while he got the keys from the office. Feeling trapped, I went along with him at first, trying to think of a way out of this situation. My mind was working fast, trying to figure out what to do without getting hurt or being left stranded in this part of town. Not knowing the type of man he was, I was afraid to risk making him angry. I did know he expected a payback for the free drinks he had so happily supplied me with earlier at the bar.

As soon as we were in the room he was ready for bed. His kisses were making me sick and I had a bad feeling about where this was going. I needed to stall for time.

"Why don't you take a shower, sweetie?" I purred into his ear, in the sexiest voice I could muster under the circumstances. I was getting frightened and thoroughly regretted my hasty decision to go for a ride with this man on the make.

He thought a shower was a good idea and wanted me to join him. "Sure, go ahead and start without me, I'll be right in," I said, growing angrier by the minute, not only at him, but at myself as well. I was beginning to get a clear picture of the whore I had become. Even at the young age of eighteen, I'd been on and off the streets for years. I had used men as a way to survive. Now I was seeing my life with some kind of new reality, and it made me sick. I was as angry at myself as I was at this pathetic, horny victim of a midlife crisis.

Being angry at myself wasn't easy. It didn't feel good. So without any hesitation, I began to take out all my anger on him. I saw only one way out. I had to escape from this room and from my present life.

I grabbed "sweetie's" car keys, wallet, and clothes, all of which he dropped carelessly on his way to the shower. I hated him and I wanted to humiliate him. Not only was I going to steal his car, but I was also going to leave him stark naked. The picture of him reporting the theft of his car to the police with only a towel on made me smile for a few seconds. This jerk deserved my act of revenge, I told myself as I closed the door quietly behind me. The tires squealed as I burned rubber, speeding out of the motel parking lot. I never looked back.

❦

Having a car felt good, even if it wasn't mine. I headed downtown to pick up Jack. I thought it would be better than doing this alone. Jack had been telling me that if we were living in his hometown of Detroit, he would be able to get a good job. If he was working, he told me, we'd get married. So I was going to put Jack on the spot. I now had the means to get us to Detroit, and he had to put up or shut up.

I was on the edge. My life was changing drastically, moment by moment. I was now a car thief. It was the most serious thing I had ever done.

Adrenaline was pumping through my veins and I felt dizzy.

Jack didn't know I'd stolen the car. I made up a good story and he bought it. We left San Francisco within an hour of my hasty exit from the sleazy motel. We headed east, and I was beginning to be excited about the future.

⸙

We ran low on gas and out of money at about the same time. So we filled up the tank on a lonesome road in Wyoming and drove off without paying—well, we didn't have anything to pay with—and the man at the gas station was on the phone to the police before we'd been gone two minutes. Jack found out I stole the car when we were arrested in Green River, Wyoming, less than twenty-four hours out of San Francisco. The news hit him hard and I discovered at about the same instant that Jack hadn't exactly been honest with me. He was AWOL from the Navy.

I didn't think things could get much more complicated, but I was wrong. They did. Crossing state lines had made our minor joy-riding adventure into a Federal crime. I was treated like a big-time gangster. We were the most excitement the sheriff of Green River had ever encountered. He was calling me the Black Widow, since Jack told them I planned the whole thing, including his going AWOL from the Navy. The big crybaby, I thought. Why was he lying about that? Did he imagine it would make things easier on him? Or maybe he was so angry with me for taking him across country in a stolen car, he didn't care anymore about what kind of trouble I was going to be in.

The love I thought I had for Jack vanished like smoke in a hurricane. He was acting like a child and heaping lies on my side of the ledger. The sheriff's face turned a darker shade of red when he found out I had (a) stolen the car, (b) taken money, and (c) driven off from a gas station without paying. To top it all off, I didn't have a driver's license. I was in big trouble and it made this small-town sheriff's day. This was a sleepy little village and not much other than drunken Saturday night fights were usually on the menu. They were really excited; their guns were drawn.

This, I recognized, was not a good situation. I had never been in jail before. Jail? Well, actually, I was locked in a big metal cage that was bolted to the cement floor in a back room of the sheriff's office. The cage had two bunks and a dirty, smelly toilet with a sink above it. It reminded me of a very large hamster cage and I was the hamster.

After slamming the door of the cage closed behind me and locking it with a huge medieval-looking key, the sheriff left, whistling happily to himself. I thought I was alone, until I heard something rustling behind me.

I turned around and came face-to-face with the oldest Native American woman I had ever seen. She had salt-and-pepper hair, tied in a topknot, with thin wisps falling around her face. I felt her eyes burn through me like I had a high fever.

Her brownish-red skin looked pale and unhealthy in the light that shone down through the top of the cage bars. Her teeth were stained and crooked, and a few were missing. I had never been this close to a real Indian before. I was frightened and felt vulnerable, not just because she was an Indian, but because we were locked in the cage together and I had nowhere to run or to hide.

She told me to relax and sit down. Her voice had no melody or laughter in it. Just an extremely tired, flat voice.

My heart was beating fast. I did as she said, sitting on a bunk bed topped off by the dirtiest blanket and mattress I'd ever seen. If I hadn't been so nervous, I probably would never have touched that bunk, preferring to stand, sit, or lie on the floor. At least the floor was cleaner.

She asked me why I was there. She said she had never seen a young white girl in all the jails she was in before. What had I done? Killed somebody?

I told her I had stolen a car. She laughed mirthlessly and shook her head in disbelief. I told her my boyfriend and I crossed three state lines and were the Sixties version of Bonnie and Clyde. For some strange reason I felt compelled to impress her, to prove I belonged in the cage, that I had earned it. It was as if I desperately needed her approval. Her understanding and accepting me suddenly became very important. Just to impress her, I made up stories of false bravado and a criminal past.

Finally I finished my lies. "Why are you in jail?" I asked. She owed me her story, I thought, since I had shared my incredible tales of make-believe crime.

She just looked at me. Then she told me she was in jail for the same reason all Indians are in jail: being drunk and disorderly. She looked at me with eyes that the word sadness cannot begin to describe. I could see the pain and humiliation this once proud woman had suffered. I somehow sensed the past harmony and balance of the Indian people and how that harmony, now torn apart, had become a living hell.

As our eyes locked, my mind opened, allowing a glimpse of her past to come flowing into my consciousness. I felt her despair and wondered at the triviality of my having done something so stupid as stealing a car, when here was a woman aged and profoundly burdened by the white man's injustice. I blinked and the mental connection was broken.

❦

I had other problems to face. The FBI was on its way to interrogate me. The jig was up. I knew I couldn't talk my way out of this. No one lies to the FBI. I gave them eleven pages of exact details and initialed every one, signing my true confession. Having waived all my rights, I would now wait to appear before the circuit judge for sentencing.

That, as it turned out, didn't happen for three months. In the meantime, I was to be transferred to the jail in Cheyenne, the state capital. That's where the judge did his work when he was in Wyoming. Thank God, I thought. At least I wouldn't have to be stuck in this rat's cage for three months. I didn't think I could survive that.

When I was returned to the cage, the Indian woman was gone. When I asked what happened to her, the sleazy guard pretended he didn't know what I was talking about.

Years later, I wondered if she had been a helping angel, one of my spirit guides, a teacher, appearing in the image of an "old Indian woman" to start the awakening process in my life. Perhaps—perhaps not. It was a remarkable meeting, nonetheless. She had opened my mind, even if only for a few moments. It closed right back down, but the seed had been planted.

The strange events of the day hadn't come to an end, as dinner was brought to me—in a cup. Beans and bread were all stuffed together in a large tin cup. It's what they supplied my breakfast in as well, except that eggs instead of beans came with the bread. There was no lunch. I quickly lost my appetite, then reluctantly lay down on the filthy bunk.

The door of the outer room opened. I was expecting the guard to return for the dinner cup, so I was startled when I heard a younger man's voice urging me to come nearer to the bars.

I was confused and looked at him closely. He was wearing a white jump suit, not the uniform of the sheriff's I had seen earlier. He quickly explained who he was. He was a "trustee," a cousin of one of the guards, doing a weekend for having been in a bar fight. He was about twenty, close to my age.

I thought I had an ally. He did have some keys, which meant he might be able to let me out.

That wasn't the case. He told me he didn't have the key to the cage, only to the room. But he was there to help me in a different way. He told me he could get me a clean mattress and pillow and blankets, even some fresh food if I was still hungry. I thought I had been sent an angel to answer my prayers. The only catch was that I had to move up to the bars and have sex with him. If I let him have his way with me, he said, he would come back with rewards. When I refused, he promised to make the rest of my time a day-to-day hell.

He did. I wasn't able to sleep more than twenty minutes at a time before the lights came on and the door opened again. I felt I must have done something terrible in a past life to deserve this kind of treatment. I contemplated giving him what he wanted, but just being around him made me more determined not to give in. The three days I spent awaiting transfer to Cheyenne were very difficult, and I was a nervous wreck by the time the Federal marshals came to drive me to the new jail. I could only hope it would be different than this one.

⚬❧⚬

It was different. Bigger, with three sets of double bunks built into the walls, even a shower, and a table with benches to sit at. Not much else. If you showered, paper towels were supplied for drying off. This wasn't the Hilton, that's for sure. Sometimes other women were there, but few stayed more than a day or a night. I got used to the isolation and handled it by sleeping much of the time. I preferred my dreams to the reality I was living.

One night, I had gone to bed at lights-out and was alone in the cell. At first I thought I was having a nightmare. Hands were around my throat, choking me. Suddenly I realized it wasn't a dream, but a reality. Someone had come in, found me asleep, and, either because she was drunk or crazy, had decided to kill me. I fought like a wild woman, kicking and screaming for help. I couldn't see a thing. I was swinging my arms and legs wildly, connecting with her now and then by accident.

I was on a lower bunk and as soon as I felt free of her, I jumped onto the higher bunk. Sitting with my back to the wall, ready to defend myself from certain death, I waited for daylight. The matrons never responded to my screams for help. I guess they either didn't hear them or had stopped caring a long time ago. By the time the sun rose, I could hear my attacker snoring. She had fallen asleep on a lower bed on the other side of the room. My throat was black and blue and both of us had multiple scratches and bruises, but when I confronted her at breakfast, she didn't remember doing anything to me. I saw no point in telling the guards. She was released that afternoon anyway.

From then on I lay on the top bunk and never again slept soundly. Any noise startled me awake. It was as if that horny jail trustee had put a bad spell on me. For the remainder of my days and nights there, my times of deep dreaming were gone. I couldn't even think about the future. If this was a series of progressively more difficult events, I couldn't begin to think what it would be like if I did get sent to prison.

⟨❦⟩

After three months of the most terrifying isolation and treatment, I was taken to the Federal courthouse. The courtroom was filled with people, but no one I knew. Many spectators just came for the show. Apparently there wasn't much to do in the God-forsaken town. I would be happy to leave it, no matter where I was going.

My knees were knocking together as I stood in front of the judge. At my side was a man in a business suit whom I had never seen before. He said out of the side of his mouth that he was my court-appointed attorney and that I should let him do the talking. I didn't even know he was going to be there. All his presence did was to confuse me and make me more nervous. Where had this guy been when I needed to talk to someone? And now, at that moment, he was to stand beside me and take advantage of his opportunity to look good? It didn't seem fair. I was learning fast that most things aren't fair.

I didn't hear much of what was going on. I was far too nervous to hear what this lawyer and the hanging judge were saying. But when the judge announced the sentence, I paid close attention. This was about me. This was my life and what was going to be happening in that life for the next few years. I paid attention to every word.

The Federal circuit judge gave me a six-months-to-six-years sentence. This was a result of the Federal Youth Offender Act, a law designed to let the prison staff release young prisoners after they served a minimum of six months, or to hang onto them for up to six years. It all depended on the prisoner's behavior and rehabilitation.

All I heard was six years! God, I'd be an old woman of twenty-four in six years. As I was being led out of the courtroom by a stocky matron,

I started shouting, "I want to see the Attorney General." I made such a fuss that I tripped over the court stenographer, sending his recorder halfway across the floor. All the commotion and confusion focused the judge's attention back in my direction. He dismissed my case after sentencing me, whereupon, according to courtroom procedure, I should have disappeared. He was through with me, but now I became both visible and audible to him again.

"What do you want?" he asked. I told him I wanted to see the Attorney General.

"Robert Kennedy?" he asked, in an incredulous voice.

"Is he here, too?" I asked ignorantly. I had heard the term "Attorney General" while being questioned by the FBI, so I figured it was someone to whom I could make an appeal to have my sentence reduced, and I just said the first thing that popped into my mind. Desperate for help, I was asking for the highest lawyer in the land. I had no idea who the Attorney General was.

It didn't work. Shortly, I was on my way to Terminal Island, near San Pedro, in Southern California, to one of the two Federal prisons in the United States for women.

NO SUCH THING AS A FREE DRINK

2

DOING TIME

The women's prison was located in one section of a minimum-security men's prison on Terminal Island. A fence some twenty feet high separated the men's and women's sections. The fence between those two sections was actually higher than the fence separating all the prisoners from the outside world. It struck me as odd.

The Marshall, my travel escort, brought me in through the prison gates. Armed guards were clearly visible, peering down from their gun towers. My wrists were handcuffed and attached to a chain encircling my waist. This was serious. I was, after all, a car thief. I was going to do time for stealing a six-year-old Chevrolet. Was this justice?

New prisoners were placed in a small building with individual rooms for isolation purposes as well as for safety. Until we were told the rules, checked out for diseases, and inspected by the prison staff, we didn't leave the Admission and Orientation Building. That was to be my home for at least the next seven days.

After taking a shower (witnessed by women guards dressed in military-like uniforms), being searched in all body cavities for contraband, and being deloused with flea powder on all hairy areas, I was given a loose, faded-blue, worn-out cotton dress, a used cotton bra, some new underpants, and slippers. Maybe they thought we would run away if we had shoes. I was numb to the bone with embarrassment from the dehumanizing treatment. This made Green River, Wyoming, seem like Club Med.

A quiet dinner was served to me in my room— if you call a tray pushed through a narrow slot in a locked door "served"—then I made my bed. At least I had clean sheets and a clean mattress. Thank goodness. I stretched out, exhausted emotionally and physically, hoping sleep would come quickly. Maybe I would wake up and find this was all a bad dream.

Huge tears, hot and salty, began sliding down my cheeks onto the pillow. The reality, the enormity of what happened to me on my first day, began to sink in. I had been in prison for a little more than six hours, and it felt like six days. How was I going to do my time if six hours felt like six days? Then six months would be like six years and, God forbid, if I stayed for the long term, it would be like sixty years! I couldn't bear the thought of it.

When I'm unhappy, my mind usually cooks up helpful plans in logical, A-B-C order, so I started thinking in high gear. I wanted a plan. A couple of plans. And an alternative plan, just in case the first plans didn't work.

Coming up with the main plan didn't take long. I was going to escape. That, in fact, was all of the plans. Plans A through Z. I had to think of a way to get out of there. Not understanding the potential consequences, I happily drifted off to sleep, dreaming of the time I would be free—a natural reaction to the inhumane treatment I had suffered. I didn't think this should be happening to me. In my own mind, I was still a nice girl and certainly didn't deserve these prison walls.

⊙✤

When the sun came up, I had slept well and awoke in a good mood. My clever mind came to the rescue. I now had a purpose. As I was being given physical examinations, intelligence tests, and interviews by the staff so they could look me over for potential problems, I checked out the surroundings for routes of escape. I was downright cheerful and took all of the procedures as a temporary situation.

No problem. I was going to break out!

After dinner, I lay on my bed. There were no books, no magazines, nothing to distract or even entertain me. This Admission and Orientation was serious, and apparently they didn't want anyone taking time off from the business of adjusting to prison life. They couldn't shut off my imagination though.

My dreams were a strong and important

part of my life, and I could put myself in a sleep-trance any time I wanted. I could direct my dream-movie and slip away into fantasy land. I had perfected this skill during my three-month wait in that bleak, dreadful jail cell in Cheyenne. I was now an expert on self-induced entertainment.

My dream-state was suddenly interrupted by loud noises coming from outside the building. Multiple gunshots. Screams. More shouting. Repeated gunshots.

I wasn't able to look out my window; the glass was at least a foot thick, apparently the same material from which soft-drink bottles are made. The outside was dark; seeing anything was impossible. My door was locked, and though I pounded frantically on it, no one came. My mind was producing a million questions a second. Apparently, no one cared about me or cared about explaining those frightening noises.

Were we at war? Were mad killers loose? Was I in danger? I couldn't imagine what was going on. Then everything got very still for a few minutes. I had time to take a deep breath, to listen more closely, extending my awareness to hear beyond the walls that surrounded me.

I don't know how long I stood there, transfixed, listening with every part of me alert. Soon, what had happened became clear. Someone had tried to escape. They were trapped on the rocks outside the fence, perhaps even in the water. (Yes, it truly was an island, even though it was connected to the mainland by a bridge.) The guards in the gun towers spotted the person or persons trying to escape and opened fire with powerful semiautomatic weapons.

Oh, my God—shot at? For trying to escape? That possibility had not occurred to me. Reality came crashing down, as if I had been on the rocks myself, with bullets ricocheting, flying hot and fast around me. At that moment, I realized there was no escaping from here. This was for real, and I could do nothing to change any of it. I collapsed on the bed in total surrender and defeat. My plan failed even before it got out of my imagination. I had no chance of getting free of this box. I was trapped. Like a rat. Now what was I going to do?

Only one thing remained. Get with the program, learn the ropes, and do whatever was necessary to be released at the earliest possible time. Sounds easy. At least it did to me at the moment. It wasn't what I wanted, but it was my only option.

I completed the two-week processing through Admission and Orientation and was assigned my room in one of the dorms. They were actually barracks left over from World War II.

Since I was the youngest woman on the prison grounds, I got a great deal of attention from the older women. They tended to take me under their wing, so to speak. I learned right away what to do and what not to do.

There are hard-and-fast rules to follow in

prison. The guards have their set of rules, the inmates another. It's not uncommon for those rules to be in complete opposition, and following them is like trying to walk a tightrope without a net while you're wearing hiking boots. Before long, I found out just how hard it is to walk that tightrope called survival.

⁂

Everyone is assigned a job in prison. Since I could type, I was placed in the front office, working for the captain of the prison guard. She was older, a retired military woman—strict but fair. I liked her. I thought this was a good opportunity for me to demonstrate to the prison staff what a "good" person I was, so they would let me go after my initial six months.

The plan was sensible and I didn't foresee any problems with it. After all, I was not involved with the women who were on drugs, nor was I into any prison "romances." Basically, I went to work in the front office, ate, watched television, and went to sleep. The only difficult times were on the weekends, but I found that reading in my room was entertainment enough. Besides, staying there was safer than mingling with the population in the dayroom, either watching television or playing cards. The less contact I had with the inmates or guards, I figured, the better for me. Cheerfully, without complaint, I stayed in self-imposed isolation.

Everything seemed fine. Of course, everything always seems fine before it falls apart.

Simply working in the front office put me in jeopardy. I didn't realize that until a few of my fellow inmates confronted me while I was in line for lunch one afternoon. They were the hoods of the joint, the "bad girl" gang.

They wanted me to do a few favors for them: send out their personal mail, make a couple of phone calls, and check into some of the other inmates' records. I had access that permitted me to do all those things.

Wait a minute. Was I hearing this right? Was having been "good" going to bring me directly into the line of fire? I was, I realized, in danger and without a lifeline. If I did the things they wanted, I would eventually be caught, which would extend my time. On the other hand, if I went to the captain about the matter, I would probably lose more than time at the hands of the other inmates. "Snitching" is a big no-no and can result in serious bodily harm, even death.

Time wasn't in my favor, although I had about a week before the pressure would be put on me to complete the tasks I had been assigned by the bad girls. My initial reaction was just to disappear, run away, get lost. But the memory of nearby gunfire was too recent for me to seriously consider escape again.

The only answer was for me to make mistakes. I could get fired from my job. That way, I would be thought of by the prison guards as a minor screw-up and the women who were putting me in the crossfire would have to lean on someone else for their favors. No one can be perfect, right?

Making mistakes was easy while I was typing and taking messages. All the things I usually handled quickly and efficiently were now bringing me criticism instead of praise. I was amazed at how stupid I could be on the job. Before long, the captain requested that I be transferred out of her office.

This was the beginning of a series of jumps from the frying pan into the fire. Trying to avoid trouble, surviving in the backward world of prison, put me in positions I normally would never have come near. I felt like a I was constantly walking on a bed of hot coals. To avoid direct confrontation, I took the safe, easy way out by regularly bringing minor disciplinary actions on myself. That way, I stayed out of "real" trouble.

After being relieved of my office duties, I was transferred to the landscape crew. This was going to be great. I could be outdoors getting some sun. Being out in the open air felt good—cutting the grass, weeding the flower beds (it was important for the women's side to look good). All was going well until I realized I was playing with fire again, without a fire extinguisher in sight.

Since the ground crew worked close to the fences, we were the internal postal service for the prison system. Packages and notes (called "kites") were constantly being thrown over the walls from outside the prison as well as from the men's side within the prison. Often those packages contained drugs or money. Just touching them was a crime, certainly more serious than stealing a cheap car. Thinking about the possible consequences I would face in my new prison job scared me.

My greatest fear was that I'd make a wrong move with what came over the fence and be nailed for trafficking in heroin. It was a no-win situation. I could hardly face my fellow inmates and "just say no."

Okay, back to Revised Plan A. A minor screw-up felt like the right thing. I took a walk about bed-check time. (One way to make sure all the prisoners were where they were supposed to be was to count them. Head-counts took place every four hours, day and night.)

Just before the doors to my room were locked I took that walk. I headed for a large palm tree, smack in the middle of the grounds. Sitting still at its base, I seemed to be invisible.

The alarm sounded when my absence was

noticed by the guards who were counting heads. As they ran to and fro, even passing very close to me, I realized they couldn't see me sitting so still. I was beginning to be really thrilled with this plan, enjoying the momentary freedom. I knew it was just a bit more serious than my plan to get fired from the front office, but it would certainly take me off the ground crew and, again, out of harm's way.

I don't think I would have turned myself in to the guards so soon, except that I heard one of the inmates yelling out her window. Her name was Pearl and she was in charge of the barracks. She wasn't the official head of the dorm, but we all did what she said or suffered the sometimes brutal consequences.

I heard yelling, "Grace, if you make me miss 'Peyton Place,' I'll get you." Well, that was enough. I turned myself in, with minutes to spare before the evening soap opera came on. I knew I was in trouble with the staff but, thank God, the inmates wouldn't be out to get me. They got to watch "Peyton Place" and I got what I deserved.

My punishment was thirty days of solitary confinement. I wasn't going to get an early parole—that was for sure. My counselor told me I would probably do at least half of my six years and, if I continued behaving as I had been, I would do all of them. My plan wasn't working. I was damned if I did and damned if I didn't. Getting out wasn't going to be easy. Plus, I wanted to be alive and in one piece when I got out. The fine-line game of survival gave me a really thin wire to walk on.

But I was learning about survival—survival in very unusual circumstances. Confrontation was out of the question. Life, in fact, depended upon how well I could avoid confrontation and I was becoming adept at that. I settled in and prepared to do my time. I couldn't think about the outside and I didn't have any visitors, which really helped. Doing time was easier with no visitors. They would just remind me of what I was missing.

My mom was sad I was in prison, but she had four other kids at home to worry about. She never came to see me at all. Dad didn't know what to think, except that I'd disappointed him again (the first time was when I wasn't born a boy). He never could quite make sense of me, since I didn't obey him like all the people who'd been under his command for thirty years in the military. Dad visited me once, for about fifteen minutes. The truth is, they both pretty much gave up on me after I landed in prison.

⊘✖⊘

I remember looking through the window into the visiting room one Sunday afternoon. It was the first and last time. Too painful. Here were women who would spend hours trying to make themselves look their best for their kids to come and visit. I started crying just seeing them hug and kiss as they greeted each other. Some of the women wouldn't let their children off their laps the entire time. I could understand that. I myself longed to be held, to be cared for by someone. It hurt not to be touched—to feel so alone and unloved. But I couldn't think like that. If I did, it would make me crazy.

A few of the women with children lost their kids to the prison system when they were arrested. If family members weren't available to take care of their children, the courts placed them in permanent foster homes or adoptive homes. The courts had the idea that if a woman was in jail or prison, she was automatically an unfit mother. (Women in prison face much prejudicial behavior purely because of their gender. A simple example: we were often treated like children—bad children who had "sinned.")

Sunday evenings were even more difficult. Sunday nights, no one was surprised to hear of suicide attempts. Visiting was rough on everyone. I was glad I didn't have visitors and especially glad I didn't have any children. That would have been unspeakable. I don't think I could have made it. The mothers I saw through the glass were in pain all the time. Maybe that's why so many numbed themselves before bed every night. Heroin was plentiful, or any other drug they wanted to take. If you had the contacts and the money, you could get drugs easily, since the prison is just a micro-version of the outside. Whatever goes on outside goes on inside, only under different circumstances and with different challenges.

⚜

Ellen became a friend of mine. She was in for income-tax evasion. She was middle-class and in constant shock about being in prison. She never did adjust to it. Every Sunday her mother brought Ellen's three young children to visit. Usually on Sunday evenings, after visiting hours were over, I talked with her. She had been dieting and drinking tons of coffee and began to look really bad. I was genuinely concerned about her. I even did a Forbidden Thing: I talked to one of the guards, asking for help for Ellen. The guard's advice to me was to mind my own business. Everyone, she said, had to do her own time in her own way.

One Sunday evening I saw Ellen go into her room. I was watching a good movie on television and decided to wait until it was over before my regular visit with her. When I finally knocked on her door, she didn't answer.

My heart started beating fast and sweat broke out on my face and hands. I was frightened. Ellen should be answering the door. I decided to go in. I saw everything clearly before I ran out of the room. Ellen had committed suicide the hard, bloody way. Wrists and throat. Blood was everywhere.

They took her body away under a covered

sheet. Her room was sealed off for investigation. After three days we were told to go in and clean it up. I refused and was sent to solitary confinement for three days. I just couldn't do it. I blamed the prison for not taking steps to prevent her death. They knew she was in trouble but didn't do anything to help her. The prison staff had, in my mind, become as dangerous as the inmates. I had to watch out on all sides now. I wasn't going to die in there.

Time passed. I'd found a safe niche. Now inmates weren't interested in what I could do for them. I was classified by the staff as a minor troublemaker. I wasn't happy but I had my moments. When I needed to interrupt the monotony, I would break a small rule to get the rush that came from sudden attention—just little things, like not making my bed or ironing my clothes. It was a game I played, waiting to be called back to my dorm to do what I'd left undone. I made the most of it—taking my time, enjoying my passive resistance.

But my little games finally came to a halt, quickly and unexpectedly. While walking back to make my bed one day, I ran into Eleanor. Eleanor was the oldest woman in the prison. She had been behind bars for twenty years and would probably die in prison. She'd been a bigtime narcotics trafficker and was given the maximum sentence, without possibility of parole. She was the Boss. Eleanor made all of us toe the line.

She stopped directly in my path. My first instinct was to go around her. She moved with me. Whoops. What had I done now? Suddenly I was nervous, swallowing hard.

"What's happening, Ellie?" I tried to sound confident.

I had run into her before, and though she never said anything, I knew she was keeping an eye on me. At least that's what I heard through the grapevine. What worried me was that I didn't know why she'd taken that special interest in me.

"What are you doing?" Eleanor became the center of my universe at the exact moment she asked me that question.

All kinds of thoughts ran through my mind. "Just doing time," was the flip answer I gave.

Wrong answer. I knew it the moment I saw her blue-grey, washed-out eyes glitter and flash. Her lips became thinner as she made them into a straight line. She sort of puffed and huffed for a second or two.

"No, Dummy. I mean, what are you going to be doing when you're my age? Where will you be?"

God, I'd never thought about that. Now, with this woman standing so close, I was looking into a time-machine mirror. All I could see was my own reflection, behind prison walls, looking grey, wrinkled, and tired. I knew instantly and clearly I didn't want that!

I got the picture. I absorbed it, digested it,

and spit it out as if it were poison. That's what my life would have been—poison, a no-life, anti-life life. I had been playing the game for survival in prison. I had forgotten the possibility of life outside these walls. Eleanor brought me back to my future. Thanks to a hardened convict, I was able to turn my life around in just about five seconds.

Eleanor probably died in prison. I don't know if she deserved it or not. I'm not the judge. I do hope she cleaned up some of her karma by giving me the opportunity to see what I was doing. I am eternally grateful to her for that. She reminded me of that old Indian woman I met in the cage in Green River. I knew I had better start paying attention to those little gifts from the heavens. They were important lessons and I felt someone was looking out for me. That thought gave me hope.

❧

Getting on the good side of the prison staff was easy. I just started making my bed, ironing my clothes, and even went so far as to put on makeup. I had them confused and I knew it.

My good behavior paid off sooner than I expected. I was placed in the keypunch division of the prison and given training as a keypunch operator, which meant I was learning a trade that would make me good money on the outside. Then something entirely unexpected came along.

Politics plays an important role in Federal institutions. The Assistant Warden was an ambitious politician who saw her job as a steppingstone to greater things. So when a new Federal regulation came down the road, she wanted its implementation to be smooth as glass. That would give her an edge.

The new regulation created what was called the Work Furlough Program. It was the brainchild of some psychologists and criminologists. The theory was that everyone would benefit if certain convicts—those who were truth-worthy or knew how to do something worthwhile or were close to completing their sentences—could work in the community during the day then return to prison at night.

I was the first person picked for the program, not because I was a model prisoner (although I got my act together after my lesson from Eleanor), but because I could type. I had what they called job skills. I was employable. Also, it didn't hurt that I wasn't a dope addict.

I had mixed emotions about the privilege of going out to work during the day and coming back to sleep in prison. It wouldn't be a piece of cake—I knew that—and the risk factor of screwing up was very high. I would be tempted, very tempted. And, to be honest, I didn't know if I could stand up to the test. But what the heck? I wanted out, even if for just a few hours a day.

The first such day I was up at four in the morning. We had to leave by five to catch the bus across the bridge to the mainland. I was excited! It was a combination of first day at school, graduation, and losing my virginity—a mixture of fear, excitement, and a step into the unknown.

The women chosen for the Work Furlough Program were segregated from the main population of women so they couldn't bring contraband in or out. Prison officials had cleverly thought of that all by themselves. Thank goodness, because at least I didn't have to worry about compromise and getting into deeper trouble. Nevertheless, I complained just to make it look like I missed the other women and didn't want to be singled out for special privileges. I had become an award-winning actress by that time. The survival game was getting easier.

But getting up so early and working at a low-paying job wasn't easy. I worked as a "girl Friday" for a small firm that rented construction equipment. (The boss knew I was from prison, and he was assisted financially by the government—an incentive to hire me in the first place.) Riding there on the bus took two and a half hours, and I didn't get back to my bed until after eight in the evening. Time just to shower, eat, and fall asleep. Still, it was worth it.

Besides, I was getting to know some of the guys from the men's side who had been selected to start the Men's Work Furlough Program. We belonged to an exclusive club, the first out in the United States. We had common bonds, so falling in love with Mike, one of the cutest guys out on that program, was easy. I hadn't been with a man in three years. I missed the closeness and attention a girl can only get from a guy.

We sat next to each other at the greasy spoon where he waited for his bus and I waited for my bus. Holding hands, we talked nonstop until we went our separate ways to work. On the return trip at night, our bus routes converged near the prison, and I checked out every bus that came near, looking for his curly dark hair in the window. I began to live for the precious minutes every morning when we could be together.

Our romance—that's what it turned into—was becoming more serious. We were talking about future plans; about when we would be out of prison; about marriage, family, that stuff. I was walking on air. I felt like I was getting a chance at the brass ring and my spirit guides were even slowing down the merry-go-round so I could get a solid grip on that ring. We laughed and loved each other at the bus stop five days a week. The weekends became unbearable and seemed to last forever.

Finally, after several frustrating months of seeing each other like that, Mike and I made some serious plans. We decided to call in after work and say we missed our bus connections, then tell them we'd be on the next bus. Mike told me he knew of an inexpensive hotel in central Los Angeles, very close to the bus depot, where we could have some privacy, if only for a brief time. It sounded good to me and I went along with him, blissfully happy.

Our date day came. I didn't know what to wear. I didn't know how to fix my hair. It was as if this were my wedding day. Mike and I would have at least one and a half hours of privacy. I knew we would make love. Our relationship had gone on for over three months and the time had come. We both knew it, and though I wasn't afraid, I was fearful I would disappoint the man I loved. Not since early high school had I been so flat out, pure and simple, head over heels in love.

The time we spent there was wonderful. It was as if our love transformed the tacky, cheap hotel into a palace of luxury and light. Holding each other was like having the winning lottery ticket. We were winners when we were together, not losers, not convicts, but two wonderfully in-love lovers.

The late afternoon sunlight peeked in on us, giving, I thought, its consent and understanding. I couldn't help smiling and laughing. Life was great and we were going to beat the system. The risk had been worth it and Mike wasn't disappointed with me. His tender kisses and whispers assured me over and over that he loved me more than anyone he ever loved in his whole life. I knew it was true, because it was the truth for me.

We hated to leave our love nest, but we had to catch the next bus for Terminal Island. At least we could ride there together. That was some consolation. All I wanted to do was touch him and be near him. So when the bus came to the last stop before the prison walls, we kissed, knowing we would see each other in the morning, and we said our goodbyes.

I was floating on air as I walked back into the women's side. I went into the main office, as usual, ready for the strip search, which was routine for our going out and coming back. What I wasn't prepared for was the Captain and the Lieutenant, standing to block my path, their arms folded across their chests. Their eyes were cold and hard, staring at me as if I were a bug under a microscope. This was not usual routine. Had something happened?

Yes, something had happened. Some snitch had apparently told on Mike and me. I hadn't said anything to anyone, so Mike must have talked to one of his buddies about our rendezvous. Jealously is a lousy companion, especially in prison.

I was pulled off the program that night. I never got to see Mike again or even tell him what had gone on with me. I never knew what happened to him. I was expelled from the special Work Furlough quarters and placed back into the mainstream population. I was back on the mainline. I had had a taste of freedom, self-respect, job earnings, and, most poignantly, love. Now it was all gone, worse than when I first came to prison. I had little to lose then. Now, my life seemed over.

I didn't care about anything and especially not about myself. I was beaten. They had won. I gave up and settled down to finish the balance of my sentence. I figured I would most likely end up doing the whole six years. All for stealing a car and making the mistake of driving across some state lines. If I had stayed in California, I would never have gone to prison. Invisible boundaries on a map had altered the course of my life forever. Self-pity dug its claws deep into my soul.

But I was, after all, number-one-before-anything, a survivor. Life went on. I was back working in the keypunch division of the prison. We were doing double shifts, helping out the government with all the orders it had to process for supplies going to a faraway place called Vietnam. I didn't care. I just did my twelve-hour shift and fell asleep, too exhausted to think about the pit I had fallen into.

❦

When the time came for my next annual physical examination, which is required by the government of all inmates, I had been in prison for over three years. Three months had passed since Mike and I were together. The memory was fresh and it hurt like a paper cut hurts the next day. I wasn't looking forward to the exam.

The doctor was an uncaring soul, just picking up a few extra bucks working at the prison to supplement his retirement income. He didn't even greet me, just told me to get on the table, lie back, spread my knees apart, and take a deep breath.

He was doing more than taking a deep breath when he got through. He was gasping and sputtering.

"You're pregnant!" he shouted to me. "How the hell did this happen? Haven't you been locked up in here for the last three years?"

Whoops.

He didn't know about Work Furlough. Was it true? Was I pregnant? I panicked. What would I tell my mom? We hadn't even spoken to each other in several years, but that's what went through my mind right then: what would I tell her? My second thought was, what would I tell the Warden? That hit home more closely. I pretty much knew I was in deep trouble. Now I was going to get it. I had been the first woman out on the Work Furlough program, and now I was the first one pregnant. Well, I'd always wanted to be the first, hadn't I? I was learning to be careful about what I wished for. Sometimes wishes come true. Although, to be honest, I never thought about using pregnancy as a way out. Mike used protection. I guess it didn't protect very well.

The prison staff recommended that I have an

abortion. But I didn't want an abortion. I wanted this baby. I was twenty-one years old, desperately needing to love and be loved, and I was going to keep my baby. The idea of being a single parent didn't frighten or intimidate me in the least. In fact, after the initial shock of being pregnant wore off, I began to feel so powerful, so wonderfully alive; I felt I had the courage and strength to do anything.

The Federal government can do a lot to its prison inmates, but performing an abortion on an inmate without her consent isn't one of them. I stood up to all the pressure from the staff and finally won out. The staff did, however, make me very uncomfortable—with the cold-shoulder treatment, snide remarks, and assurances that I wouldn't be excused from any of my work details just because I was going to have a baby. But I got a lot of support from my fellow inmates, who helped me with the heavy tasks like mopping and buffing the dormitory floors.

I was paroled when I was seven months pregnant. Not, in my opinion, because of merit or accomplishment or good behavior, but because they wanted to get rid of me. I was a constant testimony to their screw-up, a regular reminder of their mistake and poor judgment. My pregnancy wasn't going to help the Assistant Warden's political career one bit.

3

WOUNDED HEART

My freedom flight from Los Angeles to San Francisco took less than an hour. My parole officer was to meet me at the airport and take me to the Florence Crittenton Home for Unwed Mothers, where I would be living. As the miles went away behind me, I could feel the weight of prison life and all of its dangers slipping away. Finally, I thought, I would be able to make a life for myself—and for my child.

I had resisted the prison staff's urging for an abortion for more than one reason. I wanted this baby very much. I never felt better, stronger, or more whole in my entire life. A tremendous change came over me after I discovered I was pregnant. And this baby was all I had left from my feelings for Mike—the man I had loved, the man of whose fate I knew nothing. In fact, I never found out what happened to him.

I had someone with me now. My baby. No longer was I alone in this world. Now I could take care of someone and that someone would love me.

Dreams of being a mother out on the streets drifted in and out of my mind as I waited for the plane to land. I wondered what my parole officer would be like. I had three years to go before my sentence would be complete. In those three years, I would have to report to my parole officer on a regular basis and not get into any trouble. No problem, I smiled to myself, feeling my swollen belly. No problem at all. I was going to get a good job and take care of my baby.

Not knowing how to recognize the parole officer, I just stood outside the gateway, waiting for someone to approach me. She had my records, with pictures, so she knew what I looked like. Besides, I was the only noticeably pregnant woman to get off the plane. Easy clue.

She found me after a few minutes. We waited for the rest of the passengers to head toward the baggage claim area so we could have some privacy in our first meeting. She led me to a chair near the windows, looking at the runway. She was pleasant-looking, seemed efficient, and was very, very professional. Her suit was expensive and well-pressed. There wasn't a wrinkle on her; my homemade maternity dress looked cheap by comparison. I felt a little less than equal, and for more than one reason.

"Miss Stanton is my name and you may call me Carole. I will be your parole officer. You will be reporting to me on a weekly basis until I determine that we can go to longer reporting dates," she said.

Fine with me, since I had no intention of messing things up this time. I was going to make it and the weekly reporting wouldn't pose any problem.

"Just do as I say and keep your nose clean, Halloran, and we'll get along just fine." That seemed to be her way of saying hello.

No problem, I agreed. We walked toward the baggage claim area. Miss Stanton—well, Carole— had arranged for me to be housed in the unwed mothers' home. She had investigated and found it to be the most advanced and upbeat such place in the Bay Area. I was lucky that she had taken the time to look into the different facilities, for I later met a young pregnant girl at another home and she said it was more like prison.

The only requirement put on me was that I not tell the other residents I came from prison. Fine with me. I didn't relish the idea of everyone knowing I was an ex-convict, anyway. It didn't fit my picture of a modern single parent and working mother. At least, that's the picture of myself I had in mind.

Later, when we arrived at the home, we went into my assigned room. It was pleasant and I was beginning to feel even happier, if that was possible. I should have known better.

Carole was discussing what would be required of me when she noted that because of "special circumstances," I was required to adhere to certain verbal parole agreements as well.

Huh?

I was totally confused. What did she mean by "verbal"? All the parole agreements I knew about were written down and required signatures of the parolee and parole officer. The Feds liked to spell things out clearly. If anyone failed in the contract, usually it was the parolee, and that meant going back to prison. What could she mean by "verbal" agreement? I began to be suspicious; I tensed up as if to ward off a physical blow.

The shock of her words hit me broadside. She told me they wanted me to give my baby up for adoption! If I did not voluntarily give my baby up, I would be cited for parole violation, sent back for the remainder of my three years, and the Feds would take my baby anyway and farm her or him out to a permanent home. My baby would be taken away from me either way. And I knew they could do it, for I had seen it happen to other women in prison.

The words rang in my head. I couldn't believe what I'd heard. My world began spinning and I was getting dizzy. I wanted to get off this crazy, treacherous spinning top called the earth. I sat down, hard, on the bed. We had been standing in my new room at the unwed mothers' home. A few minutes before, it looked wonderful, cheerful, with brightly colored curtains and bedspreads. Nothing institutional-looking here. That was a relief, since I had no idea of what a place like this would be like.

Now the colors faded and the feeling of enclosing walls swept across me like a silent and overpowering fog. What my parole officer just told me took all the joy out of my life. Nothing was cheery now.

I remembered the women I had seen come into Terminal Island, pregnant. When they were due, they went out to have their babies and came back a few days later, without their bundle of joy. The sadness in some of their faces and eyes haunted me. Now I would have the same look myself.

It looked like the Warden was going to get the last word after all. My toying with the thought that I'd be the winner of the conflict was crushed by a few words. Verbal parole agreement. No way out, no appeal. I lost all my rights when I committed a Federal crime. Now, who could I turn too? No one. I was alone, alone with a baby growing dearer and dearer to me every day, with each breath I took.

The home had counseling services available for girls awaiting the birth of their babies. Some planned to keep them; others decided on adoption. The staff was great and appeared to be very nonjudgmental, whatever choice the girls made.

That made the balance of my pregnancy tolerable. Barely. But there weren't many nights I didn't cry myself to sleep, thinking of the experience of loss I was living through. I wasn't alone in my nighttime waterworks, either. Many of the other girls were crying, feeling the pain of their own situation. I just didn't think any of them had as much cause for swollen morning eyes as I did.

Keep prison a secret. I couldn't share my grief in any real or meaningful way. I had to live a lie. This circumstance felt like an awful punishment. But for what? For what? I didn't know. I didn't like it and I had no way out.

At times I thought of running away. Running and taking my baby with me. That was actually my first reaction, just as I determined to escape from prison my first night there. But now, even without gun tower, I was trapped just as totally.

❦

Running away wouldn't be fair—not fair to the baby, that is. Sure, I could have managed it somehow, but the possible danger to my unborn child was more than I was willing to risk. Besides, the Feds would eventually find me. I still trusted the government to do what they said they would do, and one of the things you learn over and over in prison is that they will catch up with you, and you will do time. I still believed it.

Remaining in that home wasn't for me, but I stayed for the sake of what had been given to me—my gift, my child. It was to be the second hardest thing I would ever do. The first was still to come. That would be when I left my child in the hospital after giving birth.

I made some wonderful friends at the home, and not all of my time was spent crying and feeling bad with them. Though I couldn't share my whole life with anyone—nobody, not even my closest friend and roommate, knew I had come from behind bars—we did develop close friendships that came from the common bond of being pregnant (which was better than the common bond of being convicts).

Some of us would take walks or go to the movies with one another, producing the amusing sight of three or four very pregnant girls waddling together down the sidewalk. We would take a long walk, then reward ourselves with a hot fudge sundae at nearby Mel's Drive Inn, on Geary, one of the most famous drive-ins in San Francisco. We were, after all, still young women, wanting to have some fun.

On one of these occasions, three of us—my roommate, another very pregnant girl, and I—decided to see Gone with the Wind. It had been re-released and was playing at the Golden Gate Theater, on a big, big screen. We loaded up with fruit juice, popcorn, and lots of Kleenex. (We all remembered crying in the past, and now, with the raging hormones of pregnancy, we knew we had to be ready for major crying jags. This was a crying movie and we were fully prepared.)

The movie was fantastic. An emotional roller coaster. I don't know if that's what brought it on, but two of us went into labor right then.

Childbirth classes at home had prepared us fully. Since we knew we were in early stages, we decided to finish watching the movie. We figured we would have plenty of time, once the movie ended, to get to the hospital.

By the time Rhett Butler was telling Scarlett he just "didn't give a damn," my roommate and I were having strong contractions, about five minutes apart. We were in advanced labor, but we had seen the entire movie! With popcorn hanging on our clothes, we made our way to the lobby, obviously in distress, and the crowd parted for us like the Red Sea moved aside for Moses.

A traffic cop was stationed outside the doors to help with the traffic jam the film created, especially around commute time. This alert and overanxious policeman took a look at the three of us, each nine months pregnant (and there is no mistaking that stage of pregnancy, whether you've been through it or not), with two of us bent over in obvious discomfort, and he panicked. He stopped all traffic, called for paramedics, fire trucks, and ambulances. My friends and I were laughing, tears running down our faces between contractions. It was quite a riot, almost literally.

We arrived in style and without delay at the University of California Medical Center, where we had been attending prenatal clinics. The nurses took one quick look at us and hauled us up to the fourth floor for delivery.

Twelve hours passed before my pain ceased, at least the physical pain of labor. There's no time to reflect during this process. You just are and you just be…be in pain, be in labor. The hospital knew I was going to give my infant up for adoption. And I had instructed them that I wanted to hold my baby upon giving birth and that I would feed it and take care of it until I left the hospital. They had advised against my doing so, but I didn't care. I loved this baby while it was inside of me and I would be damned if I would willingly pass up the opportunity to see what I had produced and let it know how much I loved it. They couldn't deny me that precious opportunity. I just wouldn't allow it.

<hr />

She entered the world on January 8, 1968. I was awake for the entire labor and delivery. Tears were streaming down my face and I was laughing at the same time. Laughing at the physical relief, but more at the miracle I had just participated in. She cried loudly and with such force that I knew she was healthy. It was the most wonderful event I had ever dreamed could happen. Here was my little girl, who had just moments before been inside me. This was a part of me, now living and breathing outside, on her own. Feelings of love and warmth flooded into every cell of my body. I wanted to hold her next to me. My arms ached to touch her, to hold her.

After the nurses cleaned her up, she was placed by my side. God, she was beautiful. Perfect. Pink and well-formed; blue, deep blue eyes; and the tiniest little nose, lips, and ears I had ever seen. She was a miracle, and clearly the most beautiful baby that had ever been born.

When they finally took her away from me, my heart broke. My parole officer came to check me out of the hospital, to make sure I left my baby. I had to be led out of the hospital because I couldn't see; my eyes were too full of tears. Other than my baby, I didn't care about anything or anyone anymore. I was trying to harden my heart. Not to think or to feel. It was the most painful thing that had ever happened to me. I had two weeks to sign the adoption papers.

To stop thinking was impossible. Though I was given shots to stop my milk from coming in, every few hours my breasts would get hard and ache. It was a constant reminder that I had a child, a child who was hungry. My body was reacting to her hunger, automatically, in spite of medicine's attempt to separate us. We were connected, and the pain and realization of that connecting force made me feel lost and terribly alone. More alone than I had ever felt in my life. I cried for the unjust and unfair world I was living in.

⁂

By the time I signed the adoption papers, my milk had dried up. My heart was indeed beginning to harden and my mind was finally numb. My parole officer acknowledged that I had cooperated and said I would probably get off parole within a year if I continued to behave myself.

What difference would that make? It wouldn't bring my baby back. Back to a mother who never wanted to let go in the first place. It was as if my child had died, because as far as the government was concerned, I did not have a baby, nor any of the feelings of love a mother has for her own flesh and blood. This wasn't punishment. This was a life sentence of grieving and sorrow. I would never be able to forget my child, and every time I saw another little baby girl, I was reminded of my own beautiful baby. I would spend years wondering how she was, if she was healthy and happy. Where was she? Did she hate me? These questions, I knew, would haunt me forever. I just knew they would never go away.

4

WAS LOST

The loud snap in my neck could mean only one thing. It was broken. Lying flat on my back in the middle of the ravine, I could see billowy clouds floating by on the blue canvas of the sky. It was so quiet, so peaceful. Nothing seemed to be stirring. The Honda trail bike that had thrown me lay cooling at my feet. Just moments before, we had been sailing along, weaving in and out of a herd of nervous, white-faced cows and zipping over the grassy hills. Trail-bike riding, before this rude interruption, was the most fun I'd had in a long time.

Lying on the ground motionless, I had time to review the past couple of years to see what led up to this moment. There was no place to go, no one to talk to. All I could do was think.

⟨❦⟩

After giving up my daughter for adoption, I settled down to a job that Carole, my parole officer, found for me. I worked, ate, slept, and watched television. That was my life. I had moments of clarity and my life reminded me a lot of how I had survived in prison. The only difference was that I could choose different foods to eat, stay out if I wanted to, and go to a movie if I was so inclined. Usually, I wasn't. My heart wasn't into fun things. I mourned the loss of my child. The pain would go away for a while and then just the glimpse of a baby, a child, or even the sight of a pregnant woman would bring it all back. Memories of my own child would flood my mind, overflowing into my eyes at the oddest times.

Something was missing in my life. My daughter. I tried not to think about her, but I was grieving. In those days, there were no afternoon talk shows on television to help me identify my emotional state—not a lot of interest in unwed, ex-con mothers who'd had their babies taken away. Besides, I didn't watch daytime TV anyhow. My parole officer wasn't the type of person I could share my feelings with. After all, she was part of the instrument of my pain. So, I existed. Day after day, I felt numb, without a way to express my sorrow. I turned it inward and lived my life like a prisoner in a free society. Self-punishment was something I knew about. I was good at it.

True to their word, the Feds released me from parole within a year of having signed away my child. It was a bittersweet reward. I didn't really appreciate it. But it did allow me to become a drifter, not having to hold down a steady job to satisfy the parole agreement.

The San Francisco Bay Area was full of flower children, all seeking love and freedom of expression. My sister Kathleen, two and a half years younger than me, was a flower child in full bloom, and I began to tag along with her. She was not only my best friend, but she was also my only friend.

At first, the prudish conditioning I picked up in prison didn't allow me to get in the flow of things. I was often amazed at how people dressed and behaved, especially that they were so casual about whom they slept with. I had actually become the perfect image of what the prison staff said was a "proper" woman, yet I was the odd person out. I didn't fit in with straight society and I wasn't completely comfortable with these hippies. But after a while, I felt as though I was beginning to fit in. I did need to adjust to a number of things. My God, my sister didn't even use underwear! I was totally shocked. It was a difficult road to travel.

Before long, however, I had thrown my bra on my funeral pyre where old-time feminine values would be sent on their way, up in smoke. Not wearing a bra meant not being tied up or restrained. It was a new freedom, a personal one, a freedom I could feel. I began to understand the hippie movement. It was letting go of anything and everything that could possibly make me a prisoner, whether of clothing, attitudes, feelings, or actions.

I was not interested in remaining a prisoner any longer—of anything.

For the first time, I began to feel really free. My despair lessened, since I could now express my feelings to people who—by and large, anyway— didn't judge me, didn't judge me for being an ex-con or an unwed mother or simply a woman with a non-ordinary past. It seemed that the old stigmas were thrown away. And since I was a certified official rebel, I was actually considered by some to be a heroine instead of a low-life loser.

Although I still didn't feel totally at home with the people or the cause, I felt that attending college and getting involved with the student movement would be good for me. I wasn't necessarily anti-war and I didn't understand the rhetoric that was being preached all around me. For instance, the Black Panther party was beginning to establish itself and to be heard. Not understanding fully what they had in mind, I felt threatened by their radical statements. Power to the people? What in the world did that mean?

Life on the outside in the late Sixties was frustrating. I was trying to find my way in a crazy maze of people who would demonstrate in the morning, get stoned in the afternoon, then make love the rest of the day. I was doing it right along with them and having fun—sometimes. But on a daily basis it didn't feel quite right. Something was still missing in me; I felt hollow and unable to become wholly involved in much of anything, politically or emotionally. I missed my baby. The place inside of me I had been trying so hard to fill with happiness was still empty. Or maybe missing my baby was just an excuse. Maybe there isn't a place inside that can be happy. Thoughts like that were painful. The American dream is to pursue happiness and I didn't want to believe it was an empty dream. I just hadn't found my happiness yet.

Sometimes at the park, where babies came with their flowerchild mothers, I caught myself looking at them, wondering, "Could you be my child?" My arms tensed up as though to reach out and hold one of those cherubs. Not doing so often took every ounce of my self-control. I was afraid I wouldn't be able to let go. Gradually, though, the ache diminished, pulling itself inside, being absorbed in a deeper storage space within my heart—but ready to be recalled at a moment's notice.

Jobs were easy to get, hard to hold. I tried them all—keypunch operator, waitress, and even live-in housekeeper. That last job was an escape from responsibility. I was tired of the hippie lifestyle and unable to find a decent place to live or a job. So I answered an advertisement for a housekeeper. Besides, I was pregnant.

Over a year had passed since my daughter was born. I was off parole. And with no one to threaten me with jail if I didn't follow their rules, what I wanted was to replace my missing baby. My situation, I found out later, was not at all unusual among women who have given a child up for adoption.

The father, a reservist in the Coast Guard, was in my life only briefly. I had given no thought to birth control. When I found out I was pregnant, I was happy. He never knew he had fathered a child and I didn't want to tell him.

⚜

The housekeeper's job, work for Al and his ten-year-old son Jimmy, was a perfect solution. Al had lost his wife about a year before, and the demand of a full-time job along with raising his son alone were more than he could handle. I felt sure I could do the job—keeping the house clean, preparing meals, taking care of Jimmy and, actually, being a surrogate mother. It was no big deal. Also, the house was beautiful and Al was going to give me his second car to drive. I lucked out. The hippie community had been too loose for me. I needed structure. I even put my bra back on.

Everything was going great—except Al wanted to date me. He knew I was pregnant but that apparently wasn't a problem to him. He wanted a girlfriend. I didn't want to get involved, but I lacked the courage to reject his advances outright. I was afraid I'd lose my job, and if he decided to dump me, I'd be homeless as well as pregnant. It was a matter of survival. And I had begun to like comfort, class, and money. He provided me with a taste of the good life and I liked it better than sleeping on the floor of a room with any number of stoned individuals. I went along with Al just enough to keep him interested, not leading him on, but not discouraging him, either. It wasn't the noblest thing I ever did, but at that time my instincts just told me to survive.

The future looked bright. My baby was due in two months; I was doing my job well and was happier than I had ever been. Then disaster struck. There's an old joke: "How do you make God laugh? Tell him your plans."

I was driving home in Al's Lincoln Continental after shopping. I never saw what hit me. To turn left, I had come to a complete stop. A drunk driver towing heavy construction equipment in back of his pickup smashed into me from behind. He never even applied his brakes. The police said it was lucky I had my seat belt on. Seat belt laws were years in the future, but I seem, occasionally anyway, to have been ahead of my time.

The policeman at the scene noticed I was pregnant and insisted that I be taken by ambulance to the nearest hospital. There, after a brief examination, I was released with the warning that I probably would have some sore muscles the next day. No bones appeared to be broken and the baby was fine. The doctor gave me a heavy sedative and told me to go right to bed. I had been lucky, he said. I followed his orders to the letter.

Almost thirteen hours passed before I was fully awake. My head felt heavy on the pillow, and when I started to move, the pain was excruciating. It felt like electric shocks. I couldn't even lift my head. All I could do was yell for help.

Al was still home and came into the room. I thought I was paralyzed. The fear that the paralysis might be permanent was overwhelming. I couldn't move. If this was so serious, then maybe my baby was hurt and the hospital just hadn't discovered it.

A doctor came over within an hour and I was diagnosed as having suffered extreme whiplash. "Give her these pills three times a day, and one during the night if she wakes up," he instructed, prescribing a strong narcotic. I was supposed to stay in bed until the pain went away.

The next month was a blur. I was heavily drugged, sleeping most of the time. My mind and body had been put on hold. I could get out of bed only to go to the bathroom. Eating was out of the question. I was barely able to get milk shakes and juices down. My life was ebbing away, and I was too out-of-it to recognize what was happening or to care. I felt that my baby was dying too. My dreams were nightmarish. Poor Al didn't know what to do for me, though he did continue to follow the doctor's instructions.

The same dream woke me every morning: the sounds of a tiny bird beating its fragile wings against the window, trying in vain to get to the world outside. It was trapped between the closed glass and the heavy velvet curtains that shut out all light. I would hear my own voice crying out for someone to free this tiny creature. My heart was breaking but my body wouldn't respond when I attempted to get out of bed and help. Years later, while studying the Hopi Indians, I realized the little bird in my dream was my baby's soul trying to escape this earthly plane.

After twenty-seven days, I was admitted to the hospital. The doctors were shocked at my appearance. I was pale and dehydrated with dark circles under my eyes. I had lost nearly thirty pounds. My blood pressure was excessively low and my iron count was in the danger zone. They could not detect the baby's heartbeat. I was, indeed, near death.

The doctor recommended immediate exploratory surgery. The only way I could sign the consent form was with a huge wavy X.

Three days later, I resurfaced in this world. My eyes, unfocused at first, fixed on a red line stretching from above my bed to somewhere on my arm. I was receiving transfusions.

The doctor looked relieved to see me awake. A big smile broke over his face as I tried to formulate words. My throat was raw, my tongue felt like it was wearing a fur coat. He knew, in spite of my incoherence, what I wanted to hear. He assured me that my baby was alive and well. I was still pregnant.

The seat belt caused serious injury in my abdomen and a leaking blood vessel had been one result. I had been slowly bleeding to death internally! The surgery repaired the damage, but my recovery was touch-and-go. I was very weak and the constant medication I'd been taking for pain hadn't helped my resistance to illness or my will to live. The car accident almost claimed two lives.

After another ten days in the hospital I was released—weak, but thrilled that my baby survived. I was now eight months pregnant. Soon I would be able to start my life over again, with my child. But two days later I started having stomach pains. My temperature was going up. I called my doctor. He told me to get back to the hospital immediately.

Now I was frightened. What was happening? I'd thought everything was all right, but it wasn't. I had an infection and all appearances indicated I was in labor as well. Would it ever stop?

The doctor wasn't optimistic about saving my child—I realized later that he was more concerned with saving my life—and I delivered a stillborn baby boy in the hospital room. The doctor told me not to look. He told me he would take care of everything. I was too weak and too upset to think about anything other than the fact that I had lost another child. I was stunned when a phone call came for me in the hospital room asking me what type of funeral arrangements I wanted to make for him. The doctor hadn't prepared me for that! I had but few options, and my son was buried as a Baby Boy Halloran—the grave in a cemetery in Petaluma, California. I've never seen the grave.

◉◈◈◉

Recovering from that experience would take a long time. I couldn't go back to work at Al's because too many reminders of plans gone awry were there. I needed to get away. I settled quickly with the insurance company, which figured the loss of a child was worth about three thousand dollars. It was a great deal of money to me, enough to help me start over somewhere else.

I rented a fancy apartment, bought a used Karman Ghia and decided to live the rich life. I didn't keep track of what I was spending because three thousand dollars seemed like all the money in the world. I went wild. Still in shock about my loss, I was trying hard to move fast and spend everything as quickly as I could.

I bought a wig and a beginner's oil painting kit, then settled into my new life. It lasted until my sister Kathleen came over for dinner one night and helped me balance my checkbook. How fast can money go? I learned that night, since I was nearly broke. The time for another change had arrived.

At my apartment building, I met a nice young couple, Leo and Sherry, who had found a house and needed someone to share the rent. It sounded perfect to me. Leo, who worked on a dairy farm, said he could get me a job. It sounded great. That is, until I started working and discovered why I never liked milk. Cows, I realized, are very stupid and very smelly. That job wasn't going to last. But until something else came my way, at least I was outdoors and earning my share of the rent. Besides, the distraction was just what I needed. If I didn't keep myself busy, I would begin to feel the old wound in my heart. I didn't know how I was going to recover.

⊛

We just finished getting the barn in order when Leo and Sherry found the boss's trail bikes and we headed for the hills. I was whooping and hollering as we rode through the herd of cattle. We enjoyed terrifying the cows with the chainsaw-like sound of the bikes' motors.

I didn't see the boulder. It must have been right in front of me, dead center. I hit it head-on and flew up and over, into the ravine. I heard a bone crack when I landed—and worse, my Levi's were pulled halfway down by the impact.

Sherry was at my side first. I told her not to move me, but to help me pull up my pants. I knew more men would be coming—and I sure didn't like the idea of being half-undressed. Besides, a cute guy might be among them and I wanted to make a good impression. Strange priorities.

Leo went to the farmhouse to call for the ambulance. We were way out in the country and the ambulance had to traverse the back roads. I lay there, waiting patiently, thinking how funny life had turned out for me. It seemed to me I was being punished, but I still didn't know why. Forty-five minutes passed before the ambulance arrived.

In the meantime, I heard cows mooing; their bells were getting louder. I realized I was lying directly on their pathway back to the barn. I couldn't believe it. After surviving the motorbike accident, I was going to be trampled to death. I was so embarrassed. What a way to die. Had I lived through so much, only to be done in by some stupid cows on their way home for dinner?

Sherry was beginning to panic. She realized she couldn't move me, and the cows were definitely heading toward us. Leo had returned by this time and helped Sherry pick up the mangled trail bike. Holding it between them, they sheltered me from the herd, waving their arms and shouting for the cows to go around us. I didn't know how dangerous those cows really were, but I thought Leo and Sherry were brave to do that, nevertheless. I was grateful to have friends like them. The cows passed on either side of us, sparing us the embarrassment of dying from multiple hoof prints.

***

My right collarbone was broken. It had snapped like a pretzel. The doctor explained that they don't set collarbones, but he would immobilize it with a strange-looking butterfly cast. Nothing to it.

A broken collar bone is very painful. After the initial shock wore off, I was back on pain medication. For the second time in a few months I was drugged most of the time...and getting worried I would become addicted. But the pain was so intense that I took the pills gratefully to get some relief.

Because I was laid up, I couldn't help with the rent. My sister Kathleen said I could stay with her. She had started working, and we moved to a low-rent residential hotel in the Tenderloin District of San Francisco, one of the worst places in town to live. Pimps, prostitutes, and drug dealers lived in the neighborhood. We had hopes of building up our fortunes and finding our right place—but later. Right now, this was all we could afford.

I hit a new low. During the past two years, I'd been unconscious most of the time. The accidents, taking narcotics, and emotional suffering had produced a zombie-like existence for me. I looked at it all—so many accidents, so many losses, so many hard times. Was I unconsciously trying to die? I didn't think I was, but in truth, I was extremely unhappy most of the time. I was a survivor, but I wasn't enjoying whatever I had survived for.

Living in the Tenderloin did not produce the kind of atmosphere that is conducive to a change of attitude. Thank goodness my sister was willing to be with me. Had I been alone in those squalid surroundings, with hookers living and working down the hall, druggies nodding out in the lobby, and people even getting shot and killed right outside the front door of the hotel, I think I would have given up completely.

Instead, Kathleen always tried to get me out to see the different places in the city. We had fun together and our laughter was contagious. We had half the hotel residents coming to visit just to see what these two looney women were laughing about. We found plenty of humor in our situation and shared it with anyone who wanted to listen. In fact, the only thing that saved me was my sense of humor. It's Irish humor.

For instance, we had a Murphy bed, the old-fashioned kind that folds up into the wall. Its mattress was ancient, forcing our backs into a posture like that of an old swaybacked horse. The headboard was a huge metal bar that hinged down flush with the mattress when the bed was folded up to fit next to the wall.

One night after giggling for hours, Kathleen and I suddenly turned over on our backs simultaneously. Wham! With a loud crack, I was struck across the forehead. I didn't say anything, because I thought someone was in the room with us and tried to knock me out. Kathleen was lying silently next to me. After what seemed like hours, I ventured a shaky, frightened whisper to her, "What the hell happened?"

"I don't know. Did someone hit you on the forehead?" she whispered back in the same tone. "Yes," I said, now more frightened than ever. I was sure a madman was in our room, planning to kill us—at least.

We lay still for another few minutes, finally realizing we were alone in the apartment. It was a one-room place, with a little kitchen and bathroom off the side. We'd pulled the bed out from the wall, settled in, and turned off the lights. No one was in the room when the lights went off and no one had come in the window or the door, the only two ways in.

We decided to turn on the light and investigate for ourselves. Upon doing so, we realized that, in turning over rapidly at exactly the same time, we had somehow shifted the balance of the bed's folding mechanism and released the metal bar of the headboard. Ordinarily it only hinges onto the mattress when the bed is tilted up and folded next to the wall. This time, however, the heavy metal bar came loose, hinged suddenly down, toward the mattress, and slammed smack into our foreheads, nearly knocking us unconscious.

Our screams of laughter woke all the neighbors on our floor. We were hysterical and couldn't stop the unrestrained peals of laughter. We had nearly been killed by our own bed. We didn't have to fear the pimps, the pushers, or the muggers, but we sure as hell had to watch out for that thirty-year-old bed.

Kathleen and I decided to go to church—partly because of our narrow escape from death's clutches and also because we heard there was a great church down the block, within walking distance. Well, we also heard if you stayed after the services, a free breakfast was provided. That sounded just right for us; in fact, too good to be true. We decided to check it out. Besides, it wouldn't hurt to thank the Big Guy for not letting us die from a bed-attack.

Glide Memorial Church was the most "happening" house of worship I ever attended in my life. The place was packed, even up in the balcony, with all kinds of people—poor, rich, black, brown, white, yellow, red. It was exciting, with rock 'n roll music instead of an organ and people jumping up from the polished wooden pews, hugging one another and singing and dancing in the aisles. I felt like Alice falling into Wonderland. What kind of church was this? People were having a good time? This wasn't the way I ever had participated in the worship of God. No one ever seemed to have a good time in any of the Catholic churches I attended in the past. My mind reeled with the possibilities of what was happening.

Then the preacher, a black man, Reverend Cecil Williams, came out to join the crowd. He had charisma, joy, and a tremendous amount of energy. He was all over the stage—singing, preaching, and making everyone feel wonderful at ten o'clock on Sunday morning. It was my kind of church!

Reverend Williams finished and ran to the exit door to greet each one of us on our way out. Not only did he say goodbye, but he also gave each of us a hug. I was a little embarrassed and actually intimidated. I wasn't used to having strangers hugging me and felt myself stiffen when he grabbed me. It was not a polite, genteel kind of hug, but an honest, powerful, engulfing bear hug. He whispered in my ear, "Why don't you go downstairs to the reception hall?"

I couldn't believe it. This preacher, whom I had just placed on a level with the saints, was coming on to me! He wanted me to go to the downstairs waiting room—for what? Him? Haw! I was getting a little uneasy about what I thought was happening.

I started to tell my sister, after she was hugged, what kind of proposition this minister had whispered in my ear, when she turned to me and said, "Why don't we go downstairs?"

What? He was telling everyone to join him downstairs? I guess I wanted to think the worst of the man who just had just taken me to a higher level of happiness and feeling of belonging than I had felt in a long time. I could see that my attitude toward men hadn't improved over the years. I still mistrusted and had little respect for them. In other words, I was ready for the Women's Movement.

Sis and I went downstairs. After all, food was waiting, and on our budget we couldn't afford to turn down anything free.

My mouth dropped open in astonishment. The reception hall was filled with people. At each wall were long tables with pamphlets and information on everything imaginable. We found the food table first. We saw the Black Panthers in one corner, talking with people who were mingling in front of their table, munching on doughnuts and sipping coffee. We saw other tables—with the literature of and representatives from various activist groups. One had a banner which caught my interest. It said "Connections." I was curious, so I wandered over, carrying my jelly doughnut.

The woman behind the counter was about my age and had long, straight, dark hair. Clearly, she wasn't wearing a bra. Her name was Kathy, and as she explained what "Connections" was, I began to get interested. She told me that men in prison seldom get to see their families because they—the men and their families—are usually poor, black, and come from the inner cities. Since most men's prisons were located out in the country, someone without a car had to depend on public transportation, which was not always available. The purpose of Connections was to provide volunteer drivers and cars to take male prisoners' families to visit.

"What about women's prisons?" An obvious challenge, it slipped out of my mouth before I could stop myself.

Her eyes became smaller and she sucked in a breath before answering me. I could see I caught her off-guard. I realized this white, upper middle-class liberal had not even considered the plight of women in prison. I was feeling smug with the notion I had one on the scoreboard, and she was losing.

She shot back at me a double-dare challenge. "Nothing, not a thing, and what are you going to do about it?"

She was clever, I had to hand her that. The doughnut suddenly didn't taste so good and I took a gulp of hot coffee to wash it down. I was confused. Suddenly I didn't feel so smug. What did she mean?

Kathy said she was plenty busy organizing for families of men prisoners, so why didn't I help her by setting up a system to provide rides for women's families?

I thought, why not? I was on unemployment, still looking for work and, to augment my share of the rent, cleaning vacant apartments in the run-down hotel where I was living. Her office, on an upper floor of Glide Church, was only a couple of blocks from my apartment. I told her I would come in Monday to see what I could do. I had no idea of the impact this chance meeting would have on my life.

Kathleen and I filled up on free food, then went back home by way of the beach, which, for those who aren't familiar with it, is nowhere near Glide Memorial Church. Kathleen liked the beach and I tagged along. We often went to see sunsets there and met a number of other people who ventured out about closing time for some sun. This had been my lucky day, I thought, as I waited for the sun to disappear. I had gone to church and, more significantly, enjoyed it. I met someone who was willing to listen to me about women in prison. And now I was watching a beautiful day come to an end. Maybe my life was going to get better. It was time for things to start going my way. This day felt like a new beginning; I was relishing its passing, actually looking forward to tomorrow.

 ⚜

Monday morning came and I was ready. I walked to Glide Church and went up the stairs to an office door marked "Connections." Kathy was sitting at a big wooden desk, talking on the phone. She motioned for me to sit down. She looked pretty organized and very serious about her work. There were other desks, though no one else was in the room. I saw many files. Rolodexes full of numbers were by the phones. This was for real. Posters depicting the struggles of political prisoners worldwide were on every wall. "Free the Brothers" and "Free the Political Prisoners" stickers were plastered over everything. I was getting nervous; this looked pretty radical, and I wasn't sure I was ready for revolutionary politics.

Kathy finished her call and we began to talk. After hearing my story, she told me I would be in charge of the newly formed Women's Division of Connections. She said she would help me, but basically I was on my own. She would show me the ropes but was too busy with the men's needs to take on any new tasks.

She was right. She was busy. The phone never stopped ringing while I was there, and when the mailman came he must have dumped over a hundred letters on the table. All of the letters were from men in prison who heard through the prison grapevine (more efficient than AT&T) about their wives or families being able to get a free ride to visit. I hadn't thought about the need before this, but I realized in an instant that I could do something to help. I would be able to give back favors that had been given to me by the few caring inmates I met during my three years inside.

The first several days were hectic. Learning where everything was in the office and how to set up a weekend visitor trip was a full-time proposition. And I had begun having headaches, which only compounded the stress. It was pounding pain, sometimes accompanied by flashing lights. I hadn't suffered many headaches in the past, so I didn't know what they were all about. But they were coming every day now. I thought I was working too hard, since I was still looking for a job and cleaning at least one filthy apartment a day. We were never home anymore; Kathleen and I would see each other only when we were going to sleep. It was an exciting and productive time for me. I just had to take more aspirin, that's all.

However, the headaches began to make my life miserable and they were getting worse. They were in full bloom even in the morning and not responding to over-the-counter assistance. I decided the time had come to go to the hospital for a checkup. After all, I had been through some serious trauma in the past several years. Maybe something was wrong. No sense taking any chances. But doing so this time was inconvenient. My life was full of productive work; I was making new friends and feeling I was worth something. Now was not the time to fall ill—not now.

Kathy understood when I told her I wouldn't be in to do my volunteer work that day.

"No problem. Call me when you get back," she said on the phone. We had become close and were working well together. She made me feel smart and able to do things I had never done before. I was grateful to her and admired her tremendously. The last thing I wanted was to bow out due to illness, but the headaches were becoming unbearable.

⚜

The doctor at the emergency room wasn't excited about my symptoms. I could see the weariness on his face; he had probably been on duty for thirty-six hours and he was exhausted. I must have sounded like a neurotic premenstrual female. He was already dismissing me, thinking of the appropriate prescription to justify his time with me.

"Did I mention the flashing lights?"

That got his attention. He immediately began a more thorough examination, starting with a visual tracking test. He asked me to follow his finger with my eyes. I couldn't do it. That, I found out a little later, was when he began thinking "brain tumor." He asked some specific questions about my headaches.

Clearly he was no longer intent on releasing me with a routine prescription. More sophisticated tests were needed, he said, as he admitted me to the hospital. I wasn't concerned—it just seemed to me they were going too far with the whole thing. The one bright spot was that because of my being unemployed and uninsured, the State of California would be picking up the tab for these tests.

After I settled into an uncomfortable standard hospital bed, a specialist came to examine me further. He seemed merely to be repeating the same tests the emergency room doctor had done only a few hours before. This was beginning to annoy me and I asked him what he was looking for.

"Well, young lady," he said briskly, "we suspect a brain tumor, but we will have to do more extensive tests either to rule it out or confirm it."

Brain tumor? I was scared to death. What did "rule out" mean? Did they really think I had one of those things? I signed the releases without even reading them. Really though, who does read the small print when faced with the possibility of being a vegetable for the rest of her life? Or dying? Not me, that's for sure.

The first test was an Arterioangiogram, a procedure in which dye would be injected into the carotid arteries, the major arteries in the neck that supply blood to the head. Then x-rays would be taken to determine whether a brain tumor was present. (This very dangerous procedure was later superseded by the CAT scan.) Although I was awake, I was nearly comatose due to the Valium flowing through my veins. The procedure was nasty. I could see, hear, and feel the pressure of the needle going into the artery in my neck, but felt no actual pain. The drugs took care of that.

Then, suddenly I felt blood gushing out of my neck. That got to me. I was petrified, and no amount of Valium could stop the adrenaline that was pumping when I saw my own blood spurting higher than the head of the doctor who was sticking me.

When they finally got the bleeding stopped, the torture really began. One at a time, my carotid arteries were injected with the dye so x-rays of my brain could be taken. The whole situation hadn't sounded good during the pre-procedure explanation and it didn't sound any better now. In fact, it was a living nightmare.

The pain was so severe, so much like fire being released into my brain, that I did the smart thing. I checked out. I went unconscious. No more pain.

The fact that I was unconscious didn't stop the doctor. He finished the test. When I woke up, a tape measure was around my neck. This was the Intensive Care Unit, where they were carefully monitoring swelling in my neck caused by internal bleeding from the carotid arteries. It seems that when the doctor stuck his needle into the arteries to inject dye for the x-ray, blood seeped into the surrounding tissue. Both arteries bled internally for a short time after the procedure. My neck measured twenty-one inches around. God, it was bigger than Scarlett O'Hara's waist in Gone with the Wind.

When your neck swells up to twice its normal size, it causes a great deal of pain and makes speech almost impossible. I could barely get out a hoarse whisper. The nurses kept telling me to keep still and not talk. Good advice, as it was too painful anyway. So many questions were forming, one after the other. Did I have a tumor? Would they have to operate, shaving my head and drilling holes in it? The nightmare wouldn't end. I couldn't ask, but I needed to know.

The result was "inconclusive." That, from the specialist on my case, was disappointing news. They hadn't found anything to indicate a tumor, but needed to do another test to further rule out the possibility. The procedure I lived through was not one hundred percent accurate. Another test, an electroencephalogram, could completely rule out the grim specter of a brain growth.

Two days later, they gave it to me, a test the Spanish Inquisitors would have been delighted to include in their array of tortures. This test was done with me sitting up, strapped into a head sling, while a doctor injected air bubbles into my spine. When the bubbles entered my brain, more pictures would be taken.

The bubble went exactly where it was supposed to go, and when it hit my brain, I left the room. Truly. My spirit went right out the top of my head. I could see myself slumped over, supported by straps, with nurses holding onto my limp arms. I was out of there. Three days passed before my eyes opened.

When I came back to my body, the doctors were waiting for me—a little herd of needle-wielding white coats—and they told me I'd failed the tests.

"Oh God," I said, "I have a tumor?" They shook their heads as if following a common point of light. Didn't I understand? I failed by not having a tumor. They went through all that work in pursuit of a tumor and I let them down.

"But what about the flashing lights? What about the headaches?" I tried to get them to give me a sensible answer. After all, I nearly died going through their tests. I needed justification for my own participation in this medical madness.

Now I heard the news: they had collectively decided I was mentally ill, that I had a deep psychological problem which was causing all the symptoms.

I was crazy? That was the answer? Well, I could believe it. I'd had all of those accidents (latent suicidal?) and—perhaps most clearly indicative of a problem—I permitted them to do those incredibly dangerous and painful tests, didn't I? That must prove how sick I really was. Which was the strange part of mental illness. You could be very sick and not know it. Now, with these learned men all in agreement, I accepted the fact that I, indeed, was over the hill, mentally defective.

An application for transfer to the psychiatric hospital was put into motion. I sank into my bed, sad, but comforted with the knowledge that at least we were going to get to the bottom of this. People do get well from mental illness, don't they? I was beginning to wonder, since I couldn't recall hearing of anyone who had recovered from a major mental problem. Maybe a brain tumor would have been better; at least it could be removed. But how do you remove mental illness?

Just to play it safe, one of the doctors decided to check one more thing before transferring me to the loony bin. My eyes. Maybe something was wrong with them that could account for the fact that they wouldn't track properly when I was given the initial neurological workup.

A specialist was called in. I was wheeled to a little closet-sized examining room and, without much of an introduction, this medical whiz began to shine a very bright light into my eyes. His nose was almost touching mine and I could smell his unpleasant breath. The brilliant illumination hurt my eyes; at the same time, my own personal flashing light show was underway in my head, looking like fireworks on the Fourth of July.

Maybe his day had not been going well. Perhaps he had been called off the golf course. For whatever reason, this doctor finished the examination within two minutes and suggested coldly that perhaps going blind would have a maturing effect on me.

Maturing effect? Well, maybe, since that simple statement aged me at least ten years. What in the world was he talking about? Going blind? What?

He told me I had retinitis pigmentosa, two Latin words that took me three days to learn to pronounce. He left with no further explanation, word of sympathy, or backward glance. My life was altered forever.

❦

The nurse wrote down the diagnosis and told me more about it as she wheeled me back to my room. The news wasn't good. Retinitis pigmentosa was a genetic disorder, with no known treatment. She indicated that the doctor said I was already legally blind and would be totally blind within a few years.

Legally blind? No known cure?

After the shock wore off, I thought maybe it was better than a brain tumor, and perhaps infinitely better than being crazy. I had already seen a lot in my young life. What else was there to see? My eyes weren't that important, were they? I really wasn't sure. It was a relief to finally have an answer, cruel as it was. Anyway, now I knew what was wrong with me. Life would be different, but at least I wouldn't be crazy or a vegetable. Just blind, that's all.

5

WAS BLIND

The cherry blossoms were in full bloom, lining the sidewalk in front of my hospital room. Those pink cotton balls, so beautiful, were swimming in front of eyes filled with tears. The shock of what the doctor told me was beginning to sink in.

February was one of my favorite months. It was the month of my birth and I loved to see the pink blossoms heralding spring in California. In a few weeks, I would be twenty-four. It felt more like sixty. I was lucky not to have a brain tumor or to be certifiably crazy. However, the fact was, I was going blind. Lucky, wasn't I? I would survive this, I told myself. I had learned certain survival skills early in my life, skills that always got me through the pain of the moment. Usually that meant burying any feeling or emotion that made me uncomfortable.

At twenty-three, I didn't realize I'd have to deal with all that pain someday. At the time, hiding it, covering it over, not feeling it, was easier. But all the anguish of the past was still there, just waiting to surface…and not necessarily when I was in a mood to deal with it.

Leaving the hospital with a pair of dark glasses, a white cane, and a prescription to learn Braille wasn't very encouraging. I went in there with a headache and left with a heartache.

My sister was not home when I returned to our apartment. I was alone in one of the seediest sections of San Francisco, which seemed fitting. This was the place to be if you were down and out. I was overwhelmed with self-pity—it was a pity party for one.

The manager of the hotel heard about my condition and invited me to dinner. I readily accepted, as I wanted to get out of the blue mood I was in and start living again.

Dinner was delicious. As I was eating, a thought began to nibble away at me. How would I eat when I was blind? What would it be like? I decided to try eating as a blind person, so I closed my eyes and, with concentration, tried to eat properly.

My host was very quiet. Finally he asked, "Just what in the world are you doing?"

My face turned red. I hadn't thought it through, since I was still acting on impulse rather than careful consideration. This wasn't the place to find out what being blind would be like. Besides, I had succeeded in getting the peas all over the table around my plate without actually having eaten many of them. I made a little mental note: when eating peas, one must use a spoon. Helpful Hint #1 for the blind.

My central sight was still good, although it also was becoming increasingly blurry. I could read, see signs in the distance, and generally tell if a man was good-looking or not. The nurse had explained that night blindness and lack of side-vision were the main problems I would experience at this stage of the eye disease. In fact, night blindness had always been a problem for everyone in my family except my father. We were the kids on the block that neighborhood children liked to play hide-and-seek with at twilight. They always wanted me to be "it," since I never could find them. At the time, it just seemed to be the luck of the draw. Now I knew it as a symptom of a disorder that would alter my life completely.

Everything began to fall into place. That's why I ran into the rock while riding the trail bike. That's why I'd sometimes stumble against curbs for no apparent reason. That's why, now and then, I'd knock over a glass at the dinner table. I had been slowly going blind, though the process occurred so slowly, I hadn't realized what was happening. Over time, my visual field narrowed like the shutter of a camera closing. I had less than five percent vision left when I was released from the hospital. The prognosis was poor.

The apartment became my cave. Acting like a wounded bear, I stayed inside for days at a time. Not knowing what to do, I called a social worker. The nurse at the hospital told me I probably would qualify for Social Security Blind Aid. I applied and discovered it was a pittance and wouldn't get me out of the low-rent district. Welfare adds insult to injury.

The only future I could possibly envision for myself was selling pencils on the corner, with my eyes lying at my feet, on a leash. It was a very bleak future, although on the bright side, I'd always wanted a dog.

Kathy, from Connections, heard about the medical diagnosis and came over from Glide Memorial Church to pull me out of my apartment. Instead of offering sympathy, she wanted to know when I was coming back to work. I couldn't believe her insensitivity. How could I work now? After all, I was going blind. That seemed to be enough of a job for anyone. My God, didn't she have any pity for me? She pointed out that, at the moment, I was not blind and I could do a great deal of work before I started selling pencils. Besides, she said, she really needed my help.

The best thing to say to people who are feeling sorry for themselves is that you really need their help. It worked for me. I went back to the office with Kathy; it was the best therapy I could have had.

I had a busy and demanding workload, setting up trips to the two women's prisons in California—the state prison in Corona and my old alma mater, the Federal prison on Terminal Island—both of which were located in Southern California. It was time for payback. Most of the staff at Terminal Island had told me I would never make it on the streets, that I would be back inside within a year. It had been almost three years now, and I was coming back—but not to stay. It was exciting for me to prove them wrong.

Setting up the trips wasn't easy for me. I remembered the sadness that imprisoned mothers felt when their children left, even though the joy of the visits outweighed the sorrow of the parting. Recalling those experiences provided me with useful guidelines.

The families I contacted about visiting were thankful to have the opportunity. Most were poor and had no transportation, no way to make such a trip. Families tend to fall apart when a member gets locked up. These visits would help keep them together and that was important.

Setting everything up among prison officials, local authorities, and family members required a lot of coordination. But with the help of three drivers, two station wagons, and a van, we headed for Southern California at six o'clock in the evening on a Friday in March (visiting was allowed only on the weekends).

With us were ten children between the ages of five and seventeen, three mothers, and two husbands. None had seen their respective family members since they went to prison. This was a very special trip, and everyone was in high spirits. After driving most of the night, we slept at a Lawyer's Guild office in Los Angeles, on couches, desks, and floors. All of us brought sleeping bags and we were happy just to have a place to rest before heading out to the prisons for visiting hours.

Getting ready in the morning reminded me of preparing for a high-school prom. They all wanted to look their best. Most of the children had never been on a long trip before and were really well-behaved, considering the circumstances. We all helped each other, making sure buttons were buttoned, zippers zipped, and lipstick put on without smudges. We were a family, bonded with the closeness of the adventure.

As we drew closer to the prison, everyone seemed to get quieter, anticipating the reunion. Seeing the prison walls was intimidating, and brought home the reality that Mommy was indeed locked up, and not away visiting a relative, going to nursing school, or whatever other fantasy had been made up to excuse the absence.

After going through the gatehouse, we went into the visitors' room. I didn't recognize any of the guards and my anticipated victorious return was beginning to sour. If no one knew who I was, what kind of impact could I make?

The mothers started coming in. I quickly forgot my personal triumph as I realized I was responsible for the joyous reunion of these women and their children. The smile on their faces and the tears of joy were payment enough. I felt I had done my part to pay back a certain debt by giving these women the opportunity to let their hearts swell with love, even if it was for only a few hours.

The first trip was a success and I began a series of regular long-distance visits on weekends. In the whole process, I accomplished a great deal and learned a lot about myself and my own abilities. Kathy, the founder of Connections, allowed me the opportunity to grow in ways I don't think I ever could have without her. I will never forget her kindness and her prompting me to try new things, to go beyond my limitations. She was a true friend and a great teacher.

Another avenue opened for me when I began speaking publicly about women's prisons and found out that people weren't shocked or turned off by my experience. They were actually interested in my story and opinions. It was a heady time for me, as these opportunities were beginning to put me in touch with a power buried deep inside me, a power that all people have but rarely get the chance to use fully.

These activities also left me little time for self-pity, though the threat of impending blindness hung like a dark cloud over my head. I could now tell I had lost a great deal of sight and my vision seemed to be getting worse. No matter how hard I tried to pretend that the physical limitations weren't there, they made their presence felt.

My love life, however, was going well. One afternoon, before I got the shocking news about my eyes, a fellow named Bill walked into our office at Connections, looking for help in finding work. He had just been released from Tracy, a prison for first-time offenders. He was good-looking and seemed very sweet. Tall, slender, with jet-black hair and to-die-for blue eyes, he was a hunk, and he put me into major shock when he asked me out for a date. My self-image had been suffering, so his attention came as a surprise. I jumped at the chance.

Before long, we decided to move in together, in an apartment near his work. He had a job at St. Mary's Hospital, which he got through our office. But we began to have difficulties living together. My classes on women's liberation weren't helpful to our relationship and actually added fuel to fire. Because Bill had been "inside," doing time, he was not in touch with the Women's Movement at all, and we argued constantly, particularly when he commented about this "broad" or that "chick."

Instinctively, I think I wanted to have a child around that time. I didn't want to marry, as I wasn't that much in love, but I did want a baby—in recognition of the fact that I'd lost two children already and wouldn't have my sight in a few years. I wanted to see my baby. Down deep, I think I also wanted to have someone who was mine, who would love me no matter what, and who would help me when I was blind. Was that selfish? I didn't know and the possibility didn't bother me. Survival instincts run deep and I just knew what I wanted. The Women's Movement also gave me the idea that I could raise a child by myself.

For me to conceive took not more than three days. Then Bill and I separated. When he later found out I was pregnant, he asked me if it was his child. I told him it wasn't. Babies had been taken away from me in the past, and I didn't want to jeopardize this one by complicating the picture through bringing a father into it—a father I didn't see a future with. It was another selfish act, born out of desperation. I would have regrets many years later, but at the time, I just wanted my baby all to myself.

So Bill never knew he had a son. Maybe someday my son will be reunited with his birth-father. Who knows?

Just about everyone advised me to get an abortion. My friends felt a child would interfere with my work, since I was now a local celebrity in the prison movement. The doctors were concerned that I would pass along the hereditary eye disorder. But no one could change my mind. I was in total denial about the possible consequences to my child. This baby was mine and there wasn't anything I wouldn't do to keep it. The baby was my ace in the hole, my secret reason for survival in the future, especially a future in which darkness was going to hold me hostage.

⁂

Giving talks about the prison experience and organizing prison visitation trips led to my having a reputation and I began receiving a great deal of mail from inmates. It was educational for me, as I was learning more about the political and socioeconomic factors associated with prisons and prisoners. I came to realize it's no accident that the majority of the prison population is poor people— whether black, brown, red, or white. The common bond among over ninety-nine percent of them is their status (well, lack of it) on the social ladder. I didn't agree with their tendency to be defensive and self-justifying, but I saw a glimmer of truth in their frustration with the system. I was becoming radicalized without even trying.

During one of my speeches, I met some Quakers, who invited me to a meeting to share my story. There, I listened to the other scheduled speaker—and that was the beginning of my education regarding Vietnam. Seeing the pictures of the devastation we caused in the countryside was an eye-opener and shocking. Before long, I was marching for peace. I felt the swell of power, not only in my belly, but in my heart and mind also. Having a say in the world events felt good.

Marching with tens of thousands of people against the war made it easy for me to believe revolution was around the corner. The hippie movement of the late Sixties had matured into an active social force. For me, there were meetings every night of the week. And classes. Natural Childbirth and Prenatal Nutrition class one evening, Women's Liberation Movement class on another. End the War class on another. With all of the possibilities, if the revolution came, and if it took form as armed insurrection as some people advocated, I wanted to be useful. I knew I would probably be blind, so I learned to break weapons down and reload them in the dark. Just in case. Personally, I hoped for a peaceful transition. It didn't make sense to me to be against war and killing, and then have to take over the government by force. I kept my thoughts to myself, as my views were in the minority among the people I was associating with.

❦

The world in which I lived during the early Seventies was exciting. Lawyers, Stanford University professors, nurses, doctors, ex-cons, writers, and even members of the Black Panther party were among my friends. I, an ex-con, unmarried and pregnant, was barely a high-school graduate, but the crowd I was in regarded those as assets, not liabilities. My self-esteem grew every day.

My daily routine became more complex during those turbulent times. My work schedule didn't slow down. I walked at least five miles every day and enjoyed life more than I ever had. I was still very much involved with Connections, setting up family visits for and corresponding with men and women in prison.

I had speaking engagements on a regular basis. Radio, newspaper, and even television interviews led to my becoming known more widely in the Bay Area. I was also a member of a cadre that marched in anti-war demonstrations. All in all, it was a full schedule. Caught up in the moment, I had no time for depression or self-pity. With all my heart, I believed the cause was just. Wanting my child not to grow up in a war-torn world gave me the drive to push on with tremendous passion.

I was fully active in the Peace Movement. My pocket was always filled with wet handkerchiefs, ready for me to don when the police TAC squad (a SWAT-like team) let go with tear gas, their weapon of choice—after the rubber bullets, that is. During the work week, when I often joined financial district commuters on the Muni Bus system, the Army surplus combat uniform I wore contrasted wildly with the double-breasted suits of the commuters who surrounded me on my way to work. Handing out leaflets, I would encourage the commuters to join our cause. Most were sympathetic and, when we ran into each other on the bus later in the afternoon, they were anxious to know how my day had gone. They were still neat and clean in their white-collar uniforms, while I would usually be sweaty, dirty, and exhausted from running up and down hills, with the police and their horses chasing us all over the place. It was a dirty job, but someone had to do it. I was, after all, working in their interest, too!

I realized after a while that I was their link to the revolution. I was also very pregnant, so I didn't think I could continue this type of participation, especially after almost getting crushed into a department store window. The TAC squad had released a barrage of tear gas over the crowd, which was centered around the St. Francis Hotel. I think President Nixon was there, along with a Vietnamese dignitary. The crowd was huge, and everyone was very angry at the people in the hotel. A group of demonstrators had successfully infiltrated the hotel and released a huge peace sign from one of the top floors. We were elated.

That's when the TAC squad fired the tear gas into the middle of the demonstrators. The crowd panicked. For safety reasons, I stayed on the fringe, near the department store. But as the crowd turned to run back, away from the spreading gas, I found myself pressed into the window. It actually buckled with the pressure of the crowd. For some unknown reason, the window didn't break, but just went with the pressure. I was very lucky that day, believing it miraculous that neither I nor my unborn child had been hurt.

I knew the time had come for me—temporarily, anyway—to hang up my marching shoes. I would concentrate on the prison visiting schedule, my prenatal classes, and learning more about raising a child alone. I had Shulamith Firestone's Dialectics of Sex, which had become my handbook on child-rearing. No Dr. Spock for me. This was going to be a political baby.

At the women's meetings, I told them my baby would be a girl and that I was going to raise her to be a totally liberated woman. We all spent hours talking about how we, ourselves, would like to have been raised. It gave me a perspective on how other women, though they had not physically been in jail, nonetheless felt like prisoners. An enlightening experience, for sure.

In fact, living in San Francisco during the early Seventies was like living in a classroom of consciousness and enlightenment. Lessons were available on every level, day and night. My luck dropped me in the middle of some of the most exciting and well-connected people I ever encountered. They were, for the most part, the movers and shakers of the revolution, and I was part of their inner circle.

⚮

My baby shower, which was held at the Connections office, was unique. The thirty-or-so people who were there talk about it to this day. Kathy and I prepared foods and borrowed two films to show. One was about a natural, home birth and the other told the story of a Guatemalan woman revolutionary fighting in that banana republic. Both were big hits. We had an avant-garde baby shower, ahead of its time, but right for our time and the types of change we were all involved in. We were blazing new trails. How could we have had a traditional baby shower and still lived with ourselves?

One of my friends, Cleo, had not shown up. A beautiful black woman and a single mother with a two-year-old son, she was my role model. I spent hours talking with her about how she was raising her son and she was an inspiration to me. I thought she was the New Woman epitomized and I wanted to be just like her. I knew she would have approved of and enjoyed the films.

Cleo did appear at the end of the party, however, and I was delighted to see her. She said she was sorry for having missed my shower, explaining that she'd just had too much to do earlier. (I already knew how busy she'd been lately—taking Spanish at the local adult educational facility, running two or three miles a day, and learning martial arts.) Then she added that she was leaving on a trip the next day, which surprised me, since I hadn't known she was thinking of going anywhere. Although curious, I was too excited about showing her my presents to pursue the matter, and we did not discuss her trip further.

The next day, I was shocked to hear on the news that Cleo, with her two-year-old son and boyfriend, had successfully hijacked a plane to Cuba! I never heard of or saw her again. Now I knew why she had been so active, learning a foreign language and getting in top physical condition. She'd been getting ready for Cuba. Cleo couldn't wait for the revolution to happen in San Francisco, so she joined one in progress.

6

SACRED VOW

The night I delivered my baby, San Francisco erupted with rain, hail, and one of the most wonderful lightning shows I had ever seen there. It was an exciting atmosphere to bring my child into.

I was well-prepared for childbirth and had Monie, my best friend, with me. She helped me through the early labor; the epidural medication helped me through the later stages. Although I felt a little guilty for doing so, I opted for pain relief. No pain was good.

When the doctor congratulated me and reported that I had given birth to a baby boy, I was totally surprised. I was sure he had made a mistake. After all of my Women's Movement classes, I was sure I was going to have a girl-child. I knew more about girls than I did about boys. Plus, I had become very radicalized in the direction of Women's Liberation (as we were calling it then), and I felt the Universe was playing a giant trick on me…giving me a boy to raise. What?

But the moment I held my son, all my doubts, all of my worries disappeared. He was beautiful and I loved him totally. Most important: no one could take this child away from me. No one. He was mine and I was ecstatic. And very tired. But I did permit them to take him to the nursery, since I was going to have my tubes tied in a few hours.

With this child, I would stop having babies. No doubt remained in my mind about the hereditary nature of RP, since, while I was pregnant, everyone in my family had been tested. Four out of the five children and my mother heard the same news I had gotten less than a year earlier. They had retinitis pigmentosa. They, too, could eventually lose their sight.

Not until the next evening—after I went through the surgery and was recovering from the anesthetic—did they bring my baby boy back from the nursery. The room was dark, and when the nurse propped me up in bed and placed my bundle of love into my arms, I asked her if she would please turn on the light.

Her sharp intake of breath warned me that something was not right. The light, she sad cautiously, was already on. I had lost all of my sight. I was totally blind. I couldn't see the baby I was holding in my arms. I held onto him with an iron grip, feeling the panic start to grasp my mind with a giant steel claw.

The nurse went for the doctor, and when both returned, they had to plead, almost force me to let go of my baby. It was difficult to believe. Was there some mistake? Had they done something in surgery to make me go blind so quickly? I hadn't been able to see my son at all! It wasn't fair, I moaned, beginning to grasp the reality. It just wasn't fair. The doctors had said I had a few years of sight left. It wasn't supposed to happen like this!

Much later, I realized that the delivery, together with the surgery that followed, stressed my eyes to their physical limit. I had been traumatized too greatly in too short a period of time. My eyes simply weren't responding to light; vision was impossible. Fortunately, a good friend who was also a nutritional counselor and who was aware of the effects of stress, started giving me super B-complex vitamins and other nutrients. Within a few days, some sight began to return and my eyes continued to improve after that. They were not as strong as they had been before I gave birth, but at least I could see my son's face, his blue smiling eyes, and his perfect little body. It was a reprieve, another chance for me, though the experience did provide a preview of what was finally going to happen, and that didn't feel good. All the practice of eating food with my eyes closed hadn't prepared me for the reality.

The temporary loss left scars and deeply buried fears. I had a taste of life without sight and it was more frightening than I had imagined. Especially when I anticipated holding a tiny infant who would be totally dependent upon me for survival during his early years. This, as usual, wasn't how I planned it.

I'd been thinking this child was going to take care of me. Now, having a closer relationship with my new friend Reality, I realized I was going to be taking care of him. My head was spinning with awareness and new insight—including, particularly, my realizing how much I loved him.

I also recognized that I had somehow held back with my daughter, knowing I would have to give her up. But with this child, I held back nothing. He was mine. Mine to take home, to keep and raise with all the love and protection I was capable of. I don't think I could have loved this baby more. And no one, least of all me, could have guessed how important he would be to me and the lessons I would learn from raising him.

⟮❧⟯

Although my sight returned, it did not come back fully. Perhaps the hormonal changes when I went from pre- to postnatal produced a lasting change that affected my eyes. And how might I have been affected by the drugs that were administered during surgery? I had no way at all of assessing that.

Kathy, my colleague from Connections, knew I felt insecure carrying my baby. So she pitched in and bought me a baby carrier and a portable playpen, and I was able to take him with me to work. I must have looked a sight, carrying a papoose on my back and tapping along with a white cane. But he could see what was going on. Everyone commented about how beautiful his eyes were and I took great pride in that. Always smiling and laughing, he was one of the happiest babies I or anyone else had ever seen. I was thrilled at his obvious good mood and healthy state. With each passing day, I loved my son more. I named him Ruchell, because it rhymed with "Michelle," the Beatles' song. We called him Ru for short.

Ru was less than a week old when I had a major speaking engagement in San Francisco. About three hundred people attended, most of whom had known Ru before he made his debut, so this was a very special event. Everyone wanted to say hello to him. Richard Hongisto, the newly elected Sheriff of San Francisco, came and patted him on his little head. My speech was on women's rights in prison and it was the beginning of a project to get equal treatment for women serving time in the city's jails. Unlike the situation in Federal prisons, women incarcerated in the city were not allowed out on work furlough, but men were. I wanted to do something about that.

My speech was well-prepared. Afterward, a number of women attorneys came up and we began to formulate a plan of action. Being involved with these people was exciting, for not only did they believe in something, but they were also able to help change the system by challenging it legally. Within the year, we had succeeded in getting a Federal judge to rule in our favor. Women serving their sentences in jail were now eligible for work furlough. We had taken on the system and won! Whoever said "You can't fight City Hall" hadn't come up against our team.

The next problem was that the majority of women who were eligible didn't have marketable job skills. In most cases, they were poor black women who had been on welfare. To survive, many had supplemented their income either with prostitution or by selling drugs. Finding employment was impossible for them. We had much work to do in order to make the victory real, and we realized the time had come to make job-skill training available to inmates, and to help provide referrals which would connect potential employers with women wanting to rehabilitate.

❦

Ru and I moved in with Kathy, who had bought a treasure, an old Victorian home near the Opera House in San Francisco. It was a huge one that survived the 1906 Earthquake and fire (rumor had it that Caruso once stayed there). We began to fill it with fellow workers, friends, and people passing through the area.

That in itself posed some unique problems for me. When people didn't understand my visual limitations, I usually ended up suffering physically in some way. They would leave a chair in the middle of the room or move other furniture, neglecting to replace it in its original position. For instance, I memorized the layout of the living room and usually walked through it to the kitchen with no problem. Unless, without warning, I fell over something that was left out of place. I ended up with a case of chronic black-and-blue shins, and was so paranoid that I tiptoed through certain areas, reaching out with my hand as Patty Duke had done when she portrayed Helen Keller. People who lived there regularly were very thoughtful, but they did make mistakes. What it all meant was this: my fading vision was definitely affecting me and I was getting progressively more afraid to venture out in the world.

Ru kept me busy and happy. In spare moments I reflected on my eye problem, but that depressed me, so I pushed those thoughts and feelings away. In their place, I came up with a Pollyanna-like optimism. Such as: maybe the original diagnosis had been in error. As though to support that possibility, a surprising and heartening development occurred.

Kathy's father, who had become a good fried, was wealthy, and he offered to send me to the world's best eye clinic, the Boston Eye and Ear Hospital. I wasn't thrilled about going through more eye examinations, but couldn't turn down what might prove to be a wonderful opportunity. I accepted. My sister Kathleen would take care of Ru, who was about nine months old now. She had become a great help, as had Kellee, my other sister, who was sixteen years younger than me. They baby-sat whenever I needed to get away for a day or two.

This trip was to take about a week and a half. I was nervous leaving Ru for that amount of time, but decided it was all right. Besides, I hadn't had a vacation in a long time, and maybe I would find out something at the world's best eye clinic. I could use some good news.

⁊⁊⁊

For three days, I commuted across Boston, from a friend's apartment to the eye clinic. They actually did have some tests I hadn't been given on the West Coast, and my spirits began to rise in spite of my past experience of hope being dashed on the rocks of reality. These tests were obviously more sophisticated than any I had been given before. Indeed, perhaps a mistake had been made in diagnosis. And who knows, perhaps a cure was available. Or at least a treatment.

I spent much time answering questions about my family's vision history. The doctor who headed the retinitis pigmentosa research department was keenly interested in the genetic aspects of the disease and I was a gold mine for him. He had a whole family to research—not only me, but also my mother, two of my sisters, and my brother, all of whom also had RP. Doctors always seemed fascinated to hear about my family tree, showing a curious but understandable mixture of sympathy for my situation along with scientific excitement at having access to such a perfect medical specimen as myself.

On the third and final day, I was scheduled to see the main doctor. I was excited. I became convinced there would be a hopeful report about my condition. Mental picture, of total cure were clear in my mind's eye.

The doctor didn't keep me in suspense for long. He barely looked up at me as I sat down in front of his desk. His white coat was unbuttoned, presenting an appearance of relaxed confidence. His glasses were sliding halfway down his nose. His grey, thinning hair fell onto his forehead. I was memorizing every detail because I knew I was going to hear something positive from this learned physician.

I couldn't have been more wrong. In a few seconds, my world came tumbling down. Not only was the diagnosis of my own forthcoming blindness correct, but my son, my precious child, would also be totally blind before he was a teenager! Of course, I knew RP was hereditary, that certain genetic tendencies existed, but totally blind? Inevitably blind? And when he was still just a child? The brutal certainty of the doctor's statement was nightmarish. I couldn't believe it. He didn't let up the attack. His next sentence literally made me topple over the back of my chair as I tried to get away from him and his harsh words. He informed me that I should never have had a child!

My vision was poor, but when my eyes filled with tears, visibility went down to zero. I must have stumbled home like a drunk, because I don't remember how I managed to get there. The doctor's words kept echoing in my brain, sending waves of pain from my head to my toes.

I wanted to scream, "No, no, not my baby!" How could this be happening? I wanted to raise my child before I lost all my sight, not to pass blindness along to the person I loved most in this world. Was God that unfair, so vengeful, that a little child would suffer? This news struck so deep that my faith in a supreme being was deeply challenged. Could a God exist that would let something like this happen?

I had to do something. That's all there was to it. I had to find a solution to this, and quickly, so I could prevent my son from going blind. I didn't give a damn about my own sight. It was my son's

I cared about now. I made a vow that evening to dedicate my life, all of my energy, to finding a solution that would allow my son to see, and to continue to see, the beauty in the world. Nothing else mattered. I would do anything to keep him in the sighted world. Nothing would get in the way of that vow. Nothing.

7

STARTING OVER

Raising Ruchell became the most important part of my life and I loved every minute of it. The radical movement lost its appeal. Ru came first.

Time passed quickly and the lessons I learned from being a mother never seemed to stop. When he was six months old, for example, he tried to feed himself, grabbing the spoon out of my hand. My immediate response was to seize the spoon and take it from his tiny fist. Then one of the first of many lightning bolts of awareness struck me like I'd been hit with a hammer.

Why not let him feed himself? It was his first noticeable act of independence, yet I tried immediately to suppress it. Was my ego so involved, so fragile, that I would lose some unknown quality of being a mother if I let this child feed himself? My son, even in his infancy, became my greatest teacher.

The mess around Ru that afternoon testified to how difficult it is to eat with utensils. He threw his spoon to the floor in a fit of frustration. Then, with a triumphant grin of satisfaction, he began eating with his hands. Of course! Isn't this the most natural way to eat? After all, I thought, by the time he is a teenager, he certainly will be using the conventional knife and fork. At six months, who needs them? Besides, he was able to feed himself, and that act was self-empowering. If my goal was to raise an independent, self-sufficient, healthy child, then I would have to learn to let go. That was, and is, the most difficult of all lessons for me to learn. Letting go.

❧

Living in a big city presented unique problems to a visually disabled mother. Before Ru could walk, I carried him on my back, papoose style, for optimum mobility and safety. This style of transportation made it easy for me to take him everywhere I went, including my new class at the Lighthouse for the Blind, two blocks away. I had begun to learn Braille, since my vision wasn't any better, and on some days I noticed it was getting worse. The only thing for me to do was learn to read with my fingertips and depend more on the white cane with a red tip, which identified me as visually impaired.

I hated the idea of displaying my limitations to the world. However, I came to understand that when one does not have good sight, functioning in the world without assistance is impossible, whether one holds onto another person or uses a cane. Little things other people took in their stride became minefields for me. Curbs were my new enemy. Without notice, I could be lying in the gutter, nursing a sprained ankle. Potholes that other people just avoided became the Grand Canyon for me. Just to survive was a daily challenge, and I often felt I was on the losing end of the battle.

My internal self-image had always been one of a person fully capable of doing and being anything. I didn't think I had any limitations, physically or mentally. Now, without sight to provide me with accurate information, I felt that self-image changing. I became more dependent. My frustration was building to the point that I felt something would soon have to blow. It wasn't depression, it was anger. Anger at the eye disease and at myself for being "handicapped."

Walking to the class was fun for Ruchell and me. While I was getting my lesson at fingertip reading, several women who worked at the Lighthouse as volunteers watched baby Ru. They were elderly blind women who had never had children, having been discouraged by family members and society from doing so because of being blind. They loved to hold and take care of a baby and were happy to play mother, even if only briefly, for an hour twice a week.

I remember the first time they had to change Ru's diaper. It was quite an experience for them, and thank goodness he was so patient and helpful.

I delighted in seeing them carefully pinning the diaper, protecting him so they wouldn't accidentally stick him with the pin. He held very still for the pinning ceremony. Maybe he knew they were doing it entirely by the "feel" method. We all breathed a sigh of relief when the deed was done. A major accomplishment.

When Ru began learning to walk, I was both terrified and proud. I was sure he would run into the street and be hurt or killed by a car. So much so that I trained him at an early age to hug the buildings as we walked on the sidewalk. I told him if he heard a car engine, he should get next to a building or some solid object, like a telephone pole or parking meter.

At that time, I ventured out only during the day. Becoming paranoid about traffic was really easy, and I realized I was jumping at loud noises more than usual. The simple fact was that now, when I was having trouble surviving on my own, I had another person dependent upon me for survival. Obviously, the time had come for us to leave the heavy traffic and crowded sidewalks. The city was no longer a fun or safe place for us to live.

But we didn't leave San Francisco for nearly six months. A nightmare was the deciding factor. I dreamed the police had surrounded the building where we lived on the third floor. Helicopters were flying overhead. A bullhorn repeatedly told us to give ourselves up. Grabbing the baby, I yelled out the window that we surrendered. The police came upstairs, fast. They handcuffed me and my roommate, hands behind our backs, while we were kneeling on the floor. Ru was crying. My concern for him was overwhelming. I told the police to take us down to Headquarters, already thinking of who to call to get us. The policeman grinned, pulled out his gun, pointed it at my head, and said, "We don't play by those rules anymore." I awakened in a cold sweat, suppressing in a scream. We moved within two weeks.

❧

My work at Connections had gone well and the organizational skills I learned there made it easy for me to train people to take over my position. I had now been out of prison for almost four years, and spent most of that time helping others, finding it deeply satisfying. Now, however, the time arrived for me to concentrate my energy on my son and myself. I'd not forgotten my vow to fight the eye disease. Not at all. The intuitive whispers were becoming loud shouts. "Leave the city, get back to nature." Those whispers became my call of the wild. I had learned to trust my intuition and now had no choice but to prepare to leave everyday civilization behind.

When Ru was eighteen months old—walking, talking, healthy, and happy—we moved to an isolated mountain community in the Santa Cruz

Mountains, some sixty miles south of San Francisco. Thus began my earth-mother, hippie-mountain-mama period. I was legally blind, which entitles me to receive monthly checks for Social Security Blind Aid and Aid to Families with Dependent Children. It wasn't a fortune and making ends meet was hard, but it was better than nothing. I didn't want to live the rest of my life unable to take full responsibility for myself and Ru, though at the moment, I just couldn't do things any better than I was doing them already.

Going from inner-city to mountaintop living was a big adjustment. Now when Ru heard a car engine, he'd have to hug a tree. My sister Kathleen helped me find a wonderful, woodsy A-frame house to rent, at the end of a mile-long dirt road. It had two-bedrooms, a loft, and a large redwood deck supported by stilts on three sides, with the mountain angling steeply downward beneath it. Two other houses were also on this particular mountaintop. Ours was between them. It was a magnificent location, though very isolated. Giant, beautiful redwood trees surrounded us. My living room view was of mountains and forests stretching off to the horizon.

Jake, the dog of all dogs, was able to stay with us. Kathleen had found him at the supermarket, waiting in a cardboard box. He turned out to be the smartest dog ever born. He sensed that I had a vision problem and quickly learned to keep out of my way. Jake usually traveled with Kathleen, but I think she left him so he could watch over the two of us. She was concerned about my ability to survive in the woods, as I had never been the outdoor type. My idea of roughing it was taking a room at Harrah's Club Hotel, overlooking Lake Tahoe. Her unease was probably justified.

Kathleen said nervously that she would stop in as frequently as she could, since she was going to college up in Marin County, about a two-hour drive from my new house. Nevertheless, we both knew it was up to me to become self-sufficient.

The challenges were not so difficult, however; they merely took ingenuity. The closest town was an hour's walk away, going downhill and two hours or more coming back, going uphill, depending on how much we were carrying. I found backpacks for all of us, including the dog. If he wanted to eat, he was going to carry his own food. We must have been a sight, the three of us, carrying packs like wilderness-bound trekkers. Once in a while, the local townsfolk offered to drive us, but we usually walked the entire way home. Couldn't complain about not getting plenty of exercise.

❧

Attention to proper nutrition became very important during my pregnancy, and teaching myself about appropriate eating turned into an ongoing educational process. It also seemed a natural place to start in my quest for better sight and for a way to prevent Ru's predicted eye problem. I read a book about biochemical individuality and how people with serious diseases could overcome their weaknesses by super-nutrition. I was not only willing to try this approach, but excited about the possibilities as well, so I stocked up on books about nutrition and vitamin therapy.

Although none of the doctors I saw ever asked what I was eating. I knew it was important. Before my initial exposure to a more healthy, balanced diet during my pregnancy, I thought fish-and-chips was a balanced meal, especially if it came with coleslaw. As a meal, it seemed to include the four food groups I memorized in my high-school nutrition class.

My master plan was to eat the most nutritious food I could, supplementing it with brewer's yeast tablets and other vitamins and minerals. Taking on the job of healthy cooking meant buying the wheat berries, grinding them to a flour, and baking my own bread. It was wonderful, but took about eight hours a day, preparing and cleaning up.

◎❦❧

We were happy living in our mountain retreat. I met our neighbors, whose households added to my ever-increasing awareness and search for knowledge. The little cabin to our left was occupied by an elderly Native American gentleman and his grandson. He frequently brought us fresh-picked

Swiss chard from his garden. He enjoyed teaching me about the earth's signs, even as his elders had shown him. Basically a city dweller, I was ignorant of nature, and my Indian friend taught me to know such things as whether the winter was going to be harsh or mild. The earth seems to plan ahead for its little creatures. If tons of nuts lay around the trees for the squirrels to stock, then it was a safe bet that a long, hard winter was on the way. If the supply was light, and if the fur on animals was thin and sparse, then a mild, short winter was inevitable. It was a wonderful learning experience for me.

The other neighbors were very interesting, also. He was a professor of entomology and she was a hippie mother. They were building, by themselves, a beautiful house and living meanwhile in a rental cottage. They were also attending one of the first courses that Werner Erhard was giving. He called it "EST" and it would later become well-known. They came back from their workshops and taught me what they learned. They were given assignments to work on until the next meeting, and I worked on them too, only I got to do it all for free.

Erhard had developed a very innovative and revolutionary type of group therapy. His approach, radical yet effective, was a course on responsibility, based on certain confrontive techniques. Even though he called everyone "assholes," people laughed and agreed. Not the usual response. The philosophy was complex and I needed years to fully understand the significance of the lessons. Nevertheless, it was a time of consciousness-raising. The neighbor on my left was teaching me earth science and Indian ways and those on my right were expanding my mind. Meanwhile I was cooking healthy meals and loving my son. Who could ask for more?

⚬⚬⚬

Ruchell loved the country. I took Shulamith Firestone's book Dialectics of Sex to heart and treated Ruchell as a little apprentice adult. Instead of buying baby toys, I gave him tools from around the house. He played in the kitchen with pots, pans, wooden spoons, and other kitchen odds and ends. He was inventive and content, not to mention noisy.

When he got a little older, I left him happily pounding away on blocks of wood with nails and a hammer. Occasionally I'd hear him hit his own fingers or hand, but he learned quickly what it felt like and self-inflicted injury usually only happened once. He never hurt himself severely and wasn't afraid to try new things. Encounters with pain simply made him more cautious.

Once when he was playing on the deck, I heard his gleeful giggles as he worked at something, pounding away industriously. Later, when I tried to take out the trash, the door seemed stuck. It wouldn't budge, no matter how hard I pushed. Ru was on the other side, laughing nonstop. He had nailed the door shut. I'd been imprisoned by an overachieving toddler. At that point I decided to abandon Shulamith and go with Legos.

⚜

It was an idyllic existence, and I finally fell in love with the quietness of the mountain country instead of fearing it, as I did at first. The relaxed atmosphere and the wonderfully satisfying foods we ate made me feel much better. I wasn't seeing better, but I was feeling stronger and healthier than I had in my entire life. It was pure bliss, being with my child and—if only through tunnel vision—watching him explore each new day as if it were a great adventure. In doing that, I myself began to see the world with renewed interest and expanded perspectives.

One afternoon, looking out the window, I noticed Ru was intently observing a blue jay on the deck railing. The bird would land, then take off as Ru approached. Ru was trying to imitate the bird's movements, flapping his little arms like wings. My initial response was to tell him he couldn't fly. Then I thought, why tell him? Maybe he could fly. As long as he wasn't placing himself in danger, why should I burst his bubble.? Let him find out for himself. He didn't get airborne that day, but at least I hadn't interfered with his learning process. Better for him to try and fail than never try at all. Besides, I believed in magic. Still do.

Often, I wondered where he was, only to have him appear in a few minutes, asking if I had called him. I always answered yes. He actually thought I had called his name out loud and I never told him I hadn't. He always contacted me, even when he got older, if I thought hard and long enough about him. In a way, I think I was developing the ability to communicate telepathically. Doing it was easy, but it never ceased to amaze me.

❧

Ru was teaching me so much, but when the rains arrived, our outdoor playtime came to an intermission. Since Northern California's rainy season is between October and April, that meant a lot of water in a relatively short time. Those gorgeous redwood trees need at least eighty inches of water a year.

Keeping my son busy and occupied became a challenge for me. Before the rains, the entire mountaintop was his playground. Now he was restricted to a small cabin. I needed to do something to prevent cabin fever. Jimmy Buffet, one of my favorite musicians, had even written a song about cabin fever, and apparently (according to the song) "shot six holes in his freezer." I sure didn't want to get that far gone. Of course, I didn't have a gun. But just hearing about the desperate act of shooting an innocent refrigerator affected me deeply. Thanks to Jimmy's clever warning, I intended to prevent the dreadful fever.

Fortunately, Ru's room was the larger of the two bedrooms. It had pine-paneled walls, with huge beams running across the ceiling. I borrowed my neighbor's drill and set to work creating an indoor playroom. I had never done anything like it before, but with the materials I collected, we set out to transform the room. When I say "we," I mean I did the work and Ru gave me instructions and a lot of lip.

I drilled holes in the beam and hung a one-man rubber inflatable raft. National Geographic magazines provided maps of the world for one wall and a multitude of natural animal pictures for the other wall. Putting my son down for his afternoon nap, to which he sometimes objected, now became quite an adventure. Along with his little pillow and favorite blanket, I placed him in his rubber raft, which floated about waist-high off the floor. I pointed out fascinating islands—like Pago Pago and Bora Bora—and other intriguing places. A little push started the raft swinging while I told him he would be sailing off to dreamland, to the islands we just located on the map. He never complained about nap time again.

Keeping the drill was a big mistake.

I found a small rocking chair that was in desperate need of repair. Instead of fixing it, I cut off the legs and rockers. That left a little seat with arms. I drilled holes in the chair and in the ceiling beam. Voila! An indoor swing. Ru loved to scare me half to death, swinging high in his room. It was wonderful. I was proud of my clever inventions.

Finally, insanity took over. I hung a rocking horse, then every piece of junk we could find or drag home.

Kathleen, when she next stopped by for a visit, was a welcome relief in our daily routine. She loved Ru's room, but made me give up the drill. I was on drill restriction. My sometimes practical sister gently pointed out that, after all, we were renting the house, and the owners probably wouldn't appreciate my making Swiss cheese out of their ceiling beams. I had to agree. Besides, there was nothing left to hang. I was finished and Ru's room was the best little playroom anyone could ever want. I was still missing my daughter, but the joy of spending so much time with Ru eased the pain. He, in turn, was well aware that somewhere he had a big sister and if we were lucky, she would find us.

Meanwhile, my sight was not improving and I was praying for guidance every night before falling asleep. I wasn't praying to any particular God, but to the Universe as a whole. I knew there was a God, but had given up on organized religion after seeing what it did to people. Catholic schools and institutions left a bad taste in my mouth.

My father and mother had me baptized when I was twelve. I resisted, to no avail. I remember telling the priest as he was making the sign of the cross on my forehead that I didn't want to be a Catholic. It did not deter him. Going to church was a constant source of contention between my father and me. Even as I got older, he would make me go with him on Sundays. One Sunday, trying my best to get out of going, I told him I didn't believe in the Catholic Church. Livid, he demanded, "If you are not Catholic, then just what the hell are you?"

Without hesitation, and just to spite him, I replied, "Buddhist."

"Spell it," he yelled in my face. I couldn't do it. He knew my weakness was spelling, and used that knowledge to his advantage. (It didn't occur to either of us at that time that I couldn't have spelled "Catholic" either.)

"If you can't spell it, then you can't be it," he said. I lost on a technicality and had to join in the Sunday ritual.

⦿⚞⦿

Now, with my eyesight failing and having heard the prophecy that my son would be totally blind before reaching his early teens, I was desperate. I knew that when I asked the Universe for help, it would respond. And so to Life, to the Universe, I prayed for guidance.

❦

A few nights later, we were invited to our neighbors' housewarming party. They had reached the point where they could camp out at their new home and were leaving the house next to mine.

Rex, my friend's husband, happened to tell us about his experience in pilot school, training in a chamber which simulated high altitude. His description of how his vision became progressively more tunneled as the available oxygen diminished was, I suddenly realized, identical to my own long-term experience of losing my sight.

Yes!

I left the party with the new information, elated. Instinctively I felt that part of my problem was a lack of oxygen to the retina and that this was causing the tunnel vision. Logic suggested that if I could increase the oxygen going to my eyes, my vision would improve. The problem was, how to do that? Breathe more? Not knowing the makeup of the cells or the physical floorplan of the body, I just didn't know what to do.

After a great deal of thinking, however, I decided to imagine getting more air into my eyes. Sitting on the deck, watching the sun set behind the range of tree-studded mountains, I imagined that air bubbles were racing to feed and nourish the back of my eyes. That didn't take long and soon my imagination was kicking into overdrive. I visualized little boats, like the ones in the pictures I had seen of Venice, with gondoliers feverishly working to bring the needed oxygen. Just thinking about the little Italian first-aid boats running up and down the capillaries was relaxing.

Visualization is now used widely in a multitude of goal-setting techniques and in numerous holistic approaches to physical well-being. At that time, however, I had never heard of it. I knew no guides or teachers to whom I could turn for help with the technique. I simply believed the mind was a powerful tool, and now I was putting that belief to the test. The statement, "I think, therefore I am," gained new meaning for me. Indeed, I realized, before any invention or work of art is brought to reality, it is first a thought. Now, as I was using imagery on a daily basis, my need to find out more about this process became a driving force in my continuing education.

Another avenue I explored came from secondhand awareness of "est". The main principle I worked with was this: we create our own world. Our problems, our successes, and our failures are all part of our consciousness. Self-responsibility is the key, an idea that was beginning to make sense to me.

For instance, people who have been diagnosed with retinitis pigmentosa were often referred to as victims. I was sure other disabilities were treated similarly, but since this one was my problem, it's what I was able to relate to. I reasoned that as long as I thought of myself as a victim, I was not going to be able to make any real changes in my sight or my life. If, on the other hand, I accepted the premise that I was responsible for what was going on with me, then what first needed changing was my attitude.

Which was not an easy thing to do. I felt much pain and confusion. Many of my old belief systems were being threatened, and accepting these new ideas seemed to involve a tremendous internal inclination to hold onto old ones. All the valuable lessons I learned from Ru, watching him develop and letting him go, would go out the window, especially when it came to something so personal and powerful as my own disease. Was I really responsible for my lack of sight? Examining my possible role in having created the illness was painful.

What could I possibly gain from having this eye problem? Good question. And attacking the people who were telling me these new ideas looked like it would be easier than trying to answer that question. They were crazy, I decided. Boy, was I attached to being right. Of course, that also meant that I was attached to being blind.

Consciousness expansion is not an easy process, but it is immensely rewarding, and in those early ears I finally learned to trust the process of change. New information became available and

I reacted to it in various ways—negatively and positively and in-between—but the point is, at least I finally allowed change to take place.

Even running away didn't help. I was told by a great teacher that once the awakening process begins, nothing can be done to reverse it. I could run away for a while, denial was an option. The path, however, was already established and my old choice was to walk on it. I soon learned, though, that many choices are available on the path. There are many crossroads and side streets on the road to enlightenment.

I began increasingly to recognize that if I were to be able to see externally, internal sight would be just as necessary. The ancient Chinese believed the blind were holy and advanced spiritual beings. They believed that by being blind, one could place one's attention more clearly on the internal vision quest. All right. I'd look inside with the idea of eventually being able to look outside.

The combination of good nutrition, visualizing increased oxygen supply to my eyes, and opening and expanding my consciousness did provide me with increased visual function. The change was subtle at first, but my field of sight was definitely expanding. Amazing. As I became aware of tangible signs of improvement, self-doubt marched in like gangbusters, and holding onto the past felt easier than jumping into the unknown.

But I had to jump anyway—if not for myself, then for Ru.

I don't think I'd have had the courage to go on the journey toward the Light only for myself. I already accepted the darkness, even found comfort in it at times. It was one of the best excuses for any and all of my failures. Who could blame a blind person? Without the fear that my son was going to lose his sight so early, I wouldn't have travelled the path I have all these years, a path strewn with pitfalls and obstacles.

However, the Universe had always been kind to me no matter how hard things seemed. It had given me my son, after all. How could I turn back on this child? I had no choice but to travel the road to alternative eye therapy. Modern medical science wrote off those with RP. I had fallen through a crack in the medical world and now had to rebuild my life myself, a life that would give me and my child hope of living normally.

After several months, I definitely regained some vision. That was real progress. I was even able to read for pleasure, sometimes consuming a book a day. My neighbors had plenty of books to lend, and they guided my selection as I increased my search for self-knowledge.

A book by Carlos Castaneda, The Teachings of Don Juan, opened my eyes to new possibilities.

Yes, opened my eyes. The author described a test that young Native American men had to complete in order to join the ranks of the elders. It was a rite of passage. They had to run across the desert on a moonless night as fast as they could. If the young men ran without tripping or stumbling, they qualified to join the tribe as adults.

At first I thought this impossible. How could anyone run at top speed, as if blindfolded, without falling? My first reaction was to dismiss it as fiction rather than truth. But as I read on, I realized that the young men placed themselves in an altered state of awareness prior to making the run. I began to envision the possibility of individuals being able to see, not with their eyes, but with their entire body, and especially with their feet. It began to make sense to me. If a young Indian was able to expand his awareness to other areas of his body, then he was most likely ready to become a man. It wasn't a magical ceremony, nor an illusion, but rather the result of an education that went beyond the physical limitations most of us accept today.

Excited about the concept, I read further. My active imagination brought the words to the motion picture screen in my mind. The sight of healthy young men running across the desert, bounding over obstacles they couldn't see, made me tingle with anticipation and hope. If these Indian youths could learn to see without their eyes, why couldn't I do the same? If it had been done before, then it surely could be done again. These were techniques others had discovered, and I was just in the process of rediscovering them!

I began to train on my own. My task was to become aware of what my feet could feel and see; it was only a matter of shifting emphasis. I began to center my awareness in the bottoms of my feet. My exposure to Braille expanded my sense of touch to a higher level of sensitivity, one that has always remained with me. Shifting the responsibility of any information-gathering sense, I realized, is purely a matter of opportunity, education, and emphasis. The process of learning to read tiny bumps with my fingertips had confirmed that to me. The sensitivity that accompanied my newfound ability was astonishing. Becoming more dependent upon the sense of touch had altered my perception and consciousness. What this brought about on an internal, spiritual level was impossible to measure.

I decided to make practical use of the idea I'd found in Castaneda's book. I determined to increase my overall awareness to include my feet. After all, feet are the primal contact with the earth, always receiving information. The signals, once interpreted, could increase my ability to get around. Thus, my feet became my early warning defense system, telling me of uneven pavement and treacherous sidewalk dips and crevices. Wearing high heels, naturally, was completely out of the question. I needed to be flat on the ground and I found that moccasins were great for giving accurate information. Of course, the best way to get in touch with what the feet read is to go barefooted. I began to do so whenever possible.

It felt good and I was really beginning to trust the information my feet provided. I no longer stubbed my toes as often, nor did I sprain my ankles on a regular basis. Often I stopped just short of a hole instead of falling into it. I gave my feet permission to do their job and, remarkably, they did it well. How logical—to compensate for poor sight by allowing all of the other senses to take over in the weak areas. Increased awareness gave me a new sense of freedom, and above all else, taught me that expanding awareness and consciousness in the physical body with inhibition is indeed possible. Learning these things and sharpening my senses took time and constant vigilance, but it was worth the work. My life got much easier and I was always in touch with the moment. If I did not pay attention, that was when I'd most likely have an accident.

STARTING OVER

8

MOUNTAIN MAGIC

Ru was growing in all the wondrous ways children do. The time we spent in the Santa Cruz Mountains was one of exploration and awakening. The bond between the two of us became stronger, laced with love, laughter, and mutual respect. The lessons we learned were intense and magical. Then came the time when moving on felt appropriate.

The isolation of the mountains began to take its toll. I was beginning to stagnate, and all this consciousness-raising was getting me a little crazy at times. I needed distractions, the kind you can only get from being in a busy, more inhabited place. It was time to move back to civilization, but not the city. Raising a child was too difficult in the city— for anyone, but especially for me.

The answer was the suburbs. I decided on Marin County, one of the most beautiful areas of Northern California. With picturesque towns like Mill Valley, Sausalito, and Tiburon overlooking the bay, it was an ideal area to live in. It was country-like, but close to the city; laid back, but infinitely more active than the mountaintop we had been living on.

My mother lived in northern Marin County, and she said we could stay with her until I found a place. Mom and I were getting along much better. I guess the old saying is true. The older I got, the smarter she got. Now a mother myself, I felt terrible for the things I put her through during my growing-up years. I prayed that my son wouldn't do to me what I did to her.

My dad died when Ru was about eighteen months old. He had been a Chief Master Sergeant in the Air Force for thirty years, a military man through and through, and I was a typical Air Force brat. He and I were always at opposite ends of the spectrum, and I had long ago given up trying to win his affection or attention. He also gave up on me about the time I first noticed boys during my freshman year in high school. I think he was always disappointed that I wasn't a boy myself and that I never quite gave him the respect he demanded and got from the men in his command.

Two weeks before he died, I went to visit him, taking Ru along for the ride. I felt the time had come for us to have a talk.

I knew he was unhappy with my lifestyle, but I also knew he wasn't going to be with us much longer, and I wanted to clear the slate. My dad was a right-wing, ex-military man, a war hero (a bombardier), and an Irish Catholic with every ounce of his being. I was an antiwar activist, ex-convict, unwed mother, member of the Socialist Party, and a Buddhist. No two people could have been more opposite, yet we were also much alike: stubborn and proud of being Irish.

He wasn't too pleased to be talking with me, but I think he also realized not much time was left. It turned out that we talked for hours. I told him I loved him and that I was very happy with my life. I was proud of my son, his grandson, and though I went against the grain of everything he stood for, I was a very happy person.

The conversation went back and forth, with neither of us justifying our beliefs, but rather trying to understand one another and what we were about. By the end of the day, two things had happened. We decided we respected each other and he got the last word in (he usually did) by saying that although he didn't approve of what I did, he would defend to the death my right to choose my own lifestyle. He was truly a fine American. I loved him that day more than I ever had. All the resentments, all the hurts were lifted, as though carried off and away in a helium balloon. I am forever grateful I followed my intuition to visit him then.

Ru somehow sensed the importance of our talk. He played in the yard almost all day, but was near enough to be attentive to everything. With only a few interruptions for food and a diaper change, he watched my father and me, and listened to us. Now, with the giant hugs between Dad and me out of the way, Ru—this little child who was not yet eighteen months old—came up to his grandfather and, without hesitation, took his hand and gently led him out the front door for a walk. It was his turn to have his grandfather all to himself.

Tears clouded my view and I watched from the window in my parents' home, seeing my son and my father walk hand-in-hand down the street. I could tell that Dad was talking to Ru, because once in a while I saw Ru look up and nod his head, as if he understood everything Dad was saying. Things couldn't have worked out better. The love my father had for me and for his grandson was finally able to flow unrestrained, without the shell he and I had both built around our hearts—a shell to protect us from the hurt we heaped so unmercifully on each other in the past.

Two weeks later, on Father's Day, my dad died. He was not quite sixty. It hurt me, but I didn't feel the guilt that usually comes with the passing of a loved one. I had been able to tell him all the things I wanted to tell him.

Ru and I, now returning from the mountaintop, moved back to my mom's house, and though that situation was only temporary, being back with the family felt good.

Before long, I found a place of my own in Novato, in the north of Marin County. It was a cute little house with a fenced back yard and a huge front yard. The rent was too high for me, as I was still on welfare, and I realized the time had come to find some roommates to lighten the financial burden.

I decided I wanted to make something of my life in the business world, to provide things I hadn't been able to afford for my son up to that time. My hippie, earth-mother, back-to-nature experiences had been very basic. Now I wanted some of life's finer things. I wanted money to spend on fun things like movies, clothes, and eating out once in a while.

I wasn't ungrateful for the lessons I learned on the mountaintop. I moved there as a pitiful, almost totally blind victim of an eye disease. When I left, I was seeing well enough to ride a bicycle. But I was still legally blind. I still had tunnel vision, though the "tunnel" had expanded slightly. I could see better at night and felt confident about getting around by myself during the day. I could see into the distance, read, and tell colors pretty well. I had difficulty with the difference among pink, lavender, and salmon—but who doesn't?

I was moving up in the world. My awareness lessons and visualizations, balanced with healthy nutrition and a deep faith and trust in the Universe and a Supreme Being, had a positive impact on me (and they do to this day). My inner being had been awakened. Now that inner being wanted to move up the ladder of success. Welfare didn't cut it anymore. I wanted to be a good provider for my son. I wanted more, much more.

I learned that California had certain services designed to help those with disabilities get educational, vocational, or job training and become fully employed and independent. Since I qualified for those services, I wanted to see what was available to me. Getting an appointment was easy, and within a few weeks I was on a job-training project—learning to do dental work. Not in the dentist's office, wearing a white lab coat, but in the dental lab, where it was hot, dusty, and above all else, extremely dangerous for a visually impaired person. Since I looked normal and could, in fact, see a little (though I had no side vision at all), my job counselor simply hadn't realized the nature of my problem, and we both got caught up in the excitement of my potential earnings. So there I was: working in a place that had plaster of Paris powder in the air, Bunsen burners on overtime at each desk station, and tiny sandpaper-tipped drills that could easily make mincemeat of fingers. Yes, it was an environment fraught with accidents waiting to happen. The money, however, would eventually be very good, especially for a single parent in the

Seventies—nearly seventeen thousand dollars a year.

Our living arrangements were settled at last. I found two roommates, Collette and Joel. Collette was a hair stylist and an accomplished stained-glass artist. Joel had completed four years in the Air Force and was doing odd jobs to supplement his income. He was a very mellow, soft-spoken guy with a lot of artistic abilities, and they made a good couple. We became friends.

Ru was respectful of their privacy and wouldn't go into their room without permission. He learned his lesson, having ventured in once before and cut his finger slightly on the glass Collette stored in their bedroom. After that, convincing Ru to stay out of their room was not hard.

There was a wonderful daycare center a few blocks from the house. Since I now had a rehabilitation training job, California State Rehabilitation helped pay for the daycare. My transportation was a bicycle, loaded with extras, including a bright yellow plastic baby seat.

The bike's regular seat was a little too high for me to ride comfortably and, not being mechanically inclined, I never adjusted it. Instead, I made a few changes. When we were coming to a stop that would require us to dismount, I gently leaned the bike all the way to the ground. Ru learned to hold himself rigid in his baby seat when I did that, not reaching out or touching the ground until I released his seatbelt. He was very clever, and while he didn't like stopping that way, he accepted my shortcomings without much complaint. He was, I think, just happy to be mobile. We covered much more territory on wheels than on foot.

After dropping Ru off at daycare, I pedaled quickly to my work training job. In spite of having bandaged cuts on every finger due to minor injuries from the sandpapered wheels, and despite having multiple burns on my arms from reaching across unseen Bunsen burners, I couldn't complain. At least I was on an upwardly-mobile track to financial stability. All of my energy and direction were motivated by my love and care for my son. His health and happiness were uppermost in my mind at all times. Being so focused, having someone to love so completely, felt good.

My vision had really improved as a result of my time in the mountain retreat. I still practiced good eating habits, although now that I was working, cooking meals from scratch wasn't practical. Still, I made quick, healthy meals from fresh foods. Daily sessions with positive visualization—pumping in oxygen—were easy to do. Time I normally wasted standing in lines or even in the shower was now therapy time, well spent. The visualization didn't take long and no tools were necessary. Just a memory. The more I remembered to do it, the better it seemed to work. I was constantly working on expanding my awareness, allowing all of my senses to be turned on.

❧

Once again, the time came to get my eyes checked. I hadn't ventured near a doctor's office since the last, emotionally draining experience. Most eye doctors, I had discovered, treat people with serious, untreatable eye diseases the same. Their callous personal manner made me feel less than human, as though I had no hope of ever achieving anything of value in my lifetime. At least that's the feeling I got during checkups with eye doctors in the past. I thought: why bother? Who needs that kind of punishment? Not me.

I would never have gone back to any doctor, but I felt glasses might help me now. I made a compromise. Instead of going to an ophthalmologist, I decided to try an optometrist. Optometrists could prescribe glasses and that's what I needed. I didn't need another lecture on retinitis pigmentosa. I felt I could write my own book on the subject.

Luck was with me. A few buildings down from work was an optometrist's office. "Yes," his receptionist said, they did accept Medi-Cal, my State medical insurance.

On the appointment day, I rushed over on a break from doing work, figuring it wouldn't take too long. I was in for one of the biggest surprises of my life.

Dr. Larry Jebrock was a Developmental Optometrist, specially trained to provide vision therapy for patients who wanted to improve their sight—not with glasses or contact lens, but through eye exercises! The exam was the most thorough test for visual function I had ever experienced.

As the doctor evaluated my ability to focus, to fuse, and to accommodate for reading, I couldn't hold back the questions that bubbled nonstop from my mouth. Dr. Jebrock took his time with me and responded to everything I asked. I was astonished when he told me that vision is a learned process and that sometimes certain abilities either aren't developed during infancy or early childhood, or are lost due to disease or trauma. The shocker was that lost abilities could be relearned through training! Why hadn't the many doctors I consulted before ever told me as much as this doctor was telling me? His concern for my visual state was real. He even asked me what I was doing to help my RP.

Did I dare share my secret eye program with this man? Checking in with my intuition, I felt I would be safe in doing so. He seemed genuinely interested. He said he believed I could do a great deal to improve my visual function with his training program. The excitement meter inside my brain was registering over the top.

That didn't last long. He said Medi-Cal wouldn't pay for the vision therapy. It would pay for a yearly exam and a pair of glasses but that was all.

Wasn't I ever going to get a break in this eye game? I had made progress on my own, but now, sitting not two feet away from me was a learned and experienced man who might help my vision, and he was out of my reach. I choked back bitter tears and asked if he gave discounts, and how much his fees were.

He said he would work out a payment plan if I drew up an agreement. Some of the words he used reminded me of the "EST" material I learned from my mountain neighbors. I boldly asked him if he had taken est. He had. We both smiled knowingly, the kind of smile that says, "Yes, you and I both know the secrets and the language." If indeed we create our environment, then I could create a way to pay for the therapy.

That evening, I pondered the day's events. I had actually met a professional who believed my case wasn't hopeless. Although he admitted he didn't know a whole lot about RP and had never worked with anyone with the problem, he was confident, based upon his thorough examination, that I could improve my visual function. My mind was on fire with possibilities. I had to figure a way to get this knowledge for myself and for Ru.

Looking at my budget and my income, I found it left little room for a payment plan. Offering him five dollars a month would be out of the question. At this stage my financial hands were tied. I was working toward having a more lucrative future, but at the moment, every penny counted. I could only offer a payment plan involving token amounts. My mind worked overtime as I slept and, to my delight, I came up with an idea when I awoke. I would offer money and I would offer my services. I had more time than money, and tons of energy.

Larry was great! He accepted my offer and took me on as his weekly cleaning lady. It should work out perfectly. I could come over after my work, when his office was closing, and give it a good general cleaning. To demonstrate my good faith and to let him judge my value and worth as a cleaning lady, I decided not to schedule time in therapy until I had cleaned the office a few times.

My first night on the job, Ru played in the reception room as I worked, happily scouring and scrubbing everything in sight. In the examination room, I polished all the shiny metal surfaces with vigor. To the mirror nailed to the wall, the one that reflected the letters—from the big E to the tiniest, almost invisible letters—I gave my best effort and attention. I scrubbed, polished, cleaned, and blew hot breath on it to bring out its sheen.

Having left a clean and shiny office behind, Ru and I walked the bike home. I couldn't see well in the dark, at least, not well enough to go fast on wheels, and certainly not with my son. We laughed and talked all the way there. More and more, Ru was becoming my night guide. He knew I couldn't see in the dark, but discovered his eyes did see in the dark. At first he thought something was wrong with him, that he wasn't supposed to see in the dark, either. It was tricky trying to explain normal and abnormal vision to a two-and-a-half-year-old. I think he got it, though, because after that discussion, whenever we walked, he took my hand and led me.

The next day, I ran over to Larry's office. Ellen, his assistant, was behind the reception desk. A few patients were in the waiting room, so I leaned over the counter and quietly asked Ellen if Larry was happy with the job I did on the office.

Her face was hard to read. She told me to wait, that the doctor would speak to me. This didn't sound good at all. Had I done something wrong? Did I miss something? Oh God, did I make sure the front door was locked tight? Had some sneaky, evil person dared to come in and steal something? Oh boy, oh boy, if someone had robbed the place, Larry probably thought I did it myself. This was bad.

My imagination, which so often is my friend, turned on me like a two-headed snake. I was sitting by the door, on the edge of my seat, measuring the distance, thinking about running back outside, never daring to come back.

Before I could dash out the door, Ellen was back, motioning me to follow her down the hall to Larry's office. He was going to talk to me in just a minute, Ellen said as she closed the door, leaving me sitting at the side of his desk.

At last Larry came in and told me everything. It turned out that my cleaning was a disaster. The mirror in his exam room, he explained, was never supposed to be touched. Apparently I had rubbed off all of its reflecting capability, making it useless. It wasn't a cheap variety, either. It was very special and very expensive. As a matter of fact, it cost as much as my therapy program would have.

Now I was in a hole I could never see myself climbing out of. I was heartbroken, but Larry was very understanding and loving. He told me not to worry. I could just pay him five dollars a month for the vision therapy, but I wouldn't be a good cleaning lady. My eyesight wasn't that great, and I don't believe he thought he could afford a visually impaired sanitary engineer anyway.

I also began to realize I would never make it at the dental lab. My skills limited me to pouring plaster molds and removing gold castings, and that wasn't where the money was. Now, with the opportunities Dr. Jebrock was offering me, I had to move on if I was going to help myself and be able to start Ru on the eye exercises—as soon as I learned them myself. The pressure I felt to prevent his becoming blind continued to motivate me.

As I entered the office of my rehabilitation counselor, my plan suddenly became boldly and brilliantly clear. I would go to college and become a scientist, specializing in nutrition and eye diseases. The picture of me sitting at a microscope, white coat on, coming up with the answer to the universal problem of blindness was certainly stirring and exciting.

My counselor sounded confused, but my determination and the wonderful benefits of my newly formed plan were indisputable to me. I got started by deciding to move to Sonoma County, which had good schools and low rent. I located the best junior college I could, discovering that rehabilitation counseling for the blind was available in nearby Santa Rosa. My still confused but willing advisor put the paperwork in motion.

❦

My eye exercises with Larry and Ellen were fantastic. Because I had moved on to the advanced stages of vision therapy, I was able to practice even the most difficult exercises and was really making progress. I even started Ru on a few simple ones, such as "palming" (covering both eyes with the palms while breathing deeply and relaxing) and eye rotation (with one eye covered and the head motionless, using the other eye to follow a penlight that's making large circles). I was learning a great deal about how the eyes work and I hungered to learn more. I was excited about the new possibilities. At times, tremendous anger flashed through me, especially when I thought of all the doctors who had been so negative, giving me little hope or anything to do that was positive. Why didn't they know what Larry knew? It just didn't seem right to me, and I wondered about the other unfortunate people who were going through the traditional medical mill, getting their emotions pulverized to globs of depressed nothingness.

We had about three months to relocate to Santa Rosa before college classes got underway. Leaving Collette and Joel was going to be difficult. We had become very close and got along beautifully. Perhaps they would move, too? I broached the subject and they seemed open to the possibility, open enough that they decided to drive up to Santa Rosa one Sunday to check out the area.

Then . . . what I heard on the phone from the emergency room almost knocked me right off my feet. Joel and Collette had been in a major car accident. Joel was in critical condition and Collette was also hospitalized. A drunk driver, in the fast lane, going about ninety miles an hour, hit their Volkswagen van from behind. The force had flipped the van end-over-front. The worse kind of accident. The other driver, a young man too drunk to be behind the wheel of anything, was essentially uninjured.

I got a neighbor to watch Ru while another friend drove me to the Community Hospital in Santa Rosa. The nurse explained that only members of the immediate family could get in to see Joel. I told her I was his sister. Well, in a way it was true. We were as close as a sister and brother. I loved him for his kindness and for his having been a great help and guide to my son, and for having been his friend.

I was hardly prepared for the sight of Joel, his head swathed in big bandages, lying still, in a coma. He had been thrown from their van and hit his head directly on the freeway's unyielding cement. Collette's injuries were less severe than Joel's, but still very serious; she had injured her back, fractured several bones, and was in a great deal of pain, emotionally and physically. She looked like someone who'd been beaten with a baseball bat. It was heartbreaking to see her in the large white hospital bed. Collette, an artist, loved colors, and the white surrounding her emphasized how pale and bruised she was. It was terrible.

At least she could talk—and she was angry. Angry at the accident and, even more, angry that the hospital staff wouldn't tell her how Joel was. I hated to tell her myself, but felt she deserved to know, since they weren't just lovers, they were best friends.

Well, Joel was hovering on the brink, in a semi-living and semi-dead state. The doctors said the next few days would be crucial. We all just had to wait and see.

For three days, I lived on hospital coffee and a few candy bars, worrying beyond any worrying I'd ever done before. Time went by slowly; hours seemed like days.

I was constantly going from the ICU, where Joel lay motionless, down the elevator to Collette's room to keep her posted. It was the most difficult job of communication I had ever attempted. I couldn't give her false hope, yet I wanted somehow to soften the reality of what I was seeing in Joel's room.

After three days, I couldn't take it any longer. But for brief minutes slumped in a lounge chair, I hadn't slept. Nor had I eaten anything but junk. I knew I was not going to be much of a help. Joel's mother, a woman I had never met and about whom Joel had not been very talkative, arrived and took charge. I could go home.

On my way out of the hospital, walking through the parking lot with a friend on the way to her car, I tripped over one of the long chunks of concrete that are planted to let drivers know where to stop when they park. What? After a moment, my thoughts came back to my own situation. My vision had gone down to near zero. I was astonished at the sudden loss of sight. Though I was too exhausted to think about it deeply, I noted two things: I was totally depressed and my vision was gone. At that moment I didn't know if it would ever come back. My best friends were severely injured, and all the progress I recently made had slipped away. Our worlds had been turned upside-down. It didn't seem fair, and the thought of trying to explain this to my little boy was beyond my comprehension. I just fell back in the car seat and started to cry. Nothing my friend said could stop the flow of tears. I was crying for Joel, for Collette, for me, and for my son. This lesson, whatever purpose it held, was a hard one to take. This was a mistake at least one of us might not live through. The Universe seemed a very treacherous and dangerous place to live in at that moment. I was not a happy individual and I wanted to scream obscenities at the moon.

MOUNTAIN MAGIC

9

SCHOOL'S IN SESSION

Some lessons are too painful. From my response to my friends' tragic accident, I learned about the degree to which stress affects eyesight, directly and undeniably. Within a few days, most of my vision had returned. Getting a good night's sleep and a couple of nutritious meals made a dramatic difference in my ability to see. The fear that all of my progress with my eyesight had been wiped out was abated for now.

The saddest part was that Joel never regained consciousness. He remained in a coma for nearly seventeen years, finally passing away in 1992. Collette needed a long, long time to heal her body, mind, and spirit. I never could begin to understand why he left us that way. It was so senseless.

That was Ru's first experience of losing a friend. He didn't fully comprehend what had happened to Joel and why Joel couldn't come back. He did know that when he asked about Joel, all of the adults got very sad. Soon Joel's name passed out of Ru's conversation—I think because he didn't want to cause us any more pain. Children have a very different view of life, taking each day as a whole new period of time for living. Holding onto the past is a learned, adult reaction. Ru suffered his loss, but recovered much faster than the rest of us.

A major part of my life had been on hold, waiting for Joel and Collette to heal. In the meantime, I found a place to live in Santa Rosa, a few blocks from the college. It was an affordable one-bedroom apartment in a great old house now reduced to providing rooms for students. The roof—a collection of old-style Victorian peaks called Witches' Hats—reminded us all of its once imposing and grand position in the neighborhood.

Ru was enrolled in a wonderful daycare center and I was going to be a full-time student. My dream of being a research scientist was well on its way to becoming reality.

My new rehabilitation counselor was a great guy. He was supportive and didn't burst my bubble of enthusiasm about becoming a world-renowned scientist, determined and committed to search for the cure for retinitis pigmentosa as well as all other debilitating eye diseases. Yes, my goals had expanded. Why not, I figured, find the cure for one eye disease, unlock the mystery of the eyes, then all diseases of sight could be cured. That seemed natural and logical to me.

With the cure for eye diseases under my belt, I would be a sure candidate for the Nobel Prize. Marie Curie became my role model. Reading all the books I could find about her, I got excited just thinking about the possibilities that science opened. Thoughts of Marie Curie and Albert Einstein walking together, sharing secrets of the Universe in the forest of New Hampshire, fired my imagination. I couldn't think of anything else so stimulating, so romantic. They were the perfect friends and lovers in my mind. I secretly thought to myself, why not? I could be like Marie Curie, helping the planet, and if I'm lucky, finding an Einstein of my own.

It was September 1973, and college was beginning amidst the sunshine of an Indian summer. My college entrance test scores were good in all but one area: math. The results of the math tests placed me at about sixth-grade level. Not too surprising, as the last time I was in a math class had been some thirteen years before.

Mr. Fink was our general math teacher back then. He also doubled as the typing instructor. Math and the sciences were a low priority for girls. Mr. Fink never seemed to mind when we giggled and wrote notes back and forth or even painted our nails during math. Interestingly, we could get away with it there, but never, never in his typing class! Things were all about business and professional there. No one got out of that class without typing at least forty-five words per minute, with fewer than three mistakes.

My solution now was to get a tutor in math. I began to understand that I would need a lot of it to be a scientist. I didn't understand the connection, since I was only interested in finding the cure for eye disease, not becoming a mathematical scientist. In fact, not until the first session with my tutor did I get the full picture of the role mathematics plays in science. According to my tutor, I would need at least six years of math classes. Trigonometry, calculus, algebra, logarithms, and other exotic-sounding words bounced around in my head. What? My brain couldn't believe what the tutor was telling my ears. There was no way I could complete six years of math. Even if I tried really hard. I was genetically defective when it came to math. I just didn't believe I had inherited the math gene, the one that accountants, bookkeepers, and scientists have in their blood. My monthly bank statement was and always had been a mystery to read and I never balanced my checkbook without assistance.

A few days passed before I recovered from the shock of seeing my goal of being a research scientist go down the drain of higher mathematics. But a dream early one morning helped me get over the loss. In my dream, I saw myself sitting hunched over a microscope, white coat and all. For days, my eye had been glued to the little peephole, watching what was evolving under the magnification of artificial lenses. Then, at the precise, exact moment the cure was to reveal itself, I looked up and started talking to someone else in the room, laughing and joking. By the time I put my eye back to the portal, the cure had passed by!

When I awoke, I interpreted the dream to mean that I just wasn't a quiet research type. I was a people person, preferring to chat with my peers rather than be isolated in the laboratory. It was perfectly clear to me. I needed to develop my college program in areas that would help fight blindness, but also allow me to be with people.

It wasn't the first time my dreams helped me move through rough waters.

⟐

I quickly changed my courses to nutrition, anatomy, physiology, anthropology, and health science. Not much math required in any of those. I was off the hook. The Universe was throwing me curves, but I was learning to hit them pretty well. One thing I could honestly say about my attitude and outlook on life was that I was willing to change. I always had Plans B and C, and usually X, Y, and Z waiting around. Or I could come up with them fast enough.

The college was wonderful and stimulating. It was very advanced in social programs, and even had a Women's Center, where the staff was willing to watch kids for the mothers who were attending college. Ru (who was four at the time) was happy with his daycare, though sometimes I couldn't get him to the Center on time. When that happened, he tagged along to Mommy's classes. The women instructors were very accepting, allowing Ru to sit quietly in the classroom. The anthropology professor, however—a bachelor—wouldn't tolerate having a child in his class. (What would he have done with a child prodigy?)

Ru had a great time at college. He was frequently helpful in my childhood nutrition class. One day when the instructor was talking about getting children to eat more healthy foods, Ru volunteered that kids like yogurt, especially strawberry. Everyone smiled and accepted his contribution. He wasn't shy and participated on most levels. I began to wonder about the education he was going to receive when he entered public school. Anything less than a college course might not be challenging enough for his bright, active mind.

Every Tuesday I took the bus and headed down to Dr. Jebrock's office for vision training. We established a wonderful relationship and I was madly in love with him by this time. I'm sorry to say he didn't feel the same way, but he was a source of some great dreams I had. One of my fantasies was that we would marry and travel to Africa, teaching vision therapy in Third World countries. If only a fraction of my rich fantasy life had come true, I'd have been the happiest camper on planet Earth.

Ellen, his vision therapist, became my friend as well, though I often got the feeling she was just tolerating me. I was always so chatty—my mouth never stopped. It was as if these were the only two people in the world I could talk to. Both were supportive when I shared my hopes and dreams about getting better sight and finding a way to prevent Ru from losing his. They listened and smiled, nodding with acceptance, which gave me the only encouragement I needed to continue my research into better vision.

Ellen had a fine educational background and I thought she was classy. She was a role-model for me, so her approval of what I did meant a great deal to me. But my ego was crushed one day when she actually told me I talked too much and said very little. After the initial shock and embarrassment wore off, I realized she was right. I had been a compulsive garbage mouth, saying anything that entered my mind, not bothering to sort the pearls from the trash. In retrospect, I see her bluntness as having been a gift, and to this day I am grateful. Truly, a good friend will also tell you the things you don't want to hear. Without that kind of feedback, how is one ever to get the opportunity to change for the better?

My eyes were holding their own. They were still better than when Ru was born, yet not where I wanted them to be. Nevertheless, after I started any new technique, adding it to my growing eye-related self-improvement program, I'd usually see some progress, though I ordinarily reached a plateau at which things seemed not to get any better. Nevertheless, whenever I began to see improvement, I would start Ru on the new technique. We enjoyed doing our eye exercises together.

Late one afternoon, I glanced around my room and noticed a large block of vivid colors on the wall. Suddenly, I was fully alert and curious. It was beautiful, suggesting what a rainbow would be like if it could be captured and frozen still. I had never seen a color pattern like it before and was curious as to its origin.

The wall was normally a soft white and had nothing on it. Tracking the color pattern back to its source led me to a surprise: a ten-gallon fish tank sitting in the window was in the right place at the right time. The sun's rays came in the window, continued into the tank, then emerged to be splayed onto the wall as a vivid spectrum of colors. It was like magic. The colors seemed to vibrate; they were shimmering and luminous. The space, if it had lasted, was large enough to have been framed.

Mesmerized by the color show, I felt an overwhelming urge come over me. Suppose I got in those colors and let them wash over my face? Quickly, before they disappeared, I sat on the floor, facing the fish tank. With my back to the wall, I settled into the red region of the rainbow. My entire being responded suddenly in a startling way.

I felt angry. My teeth clenched tightly together and my breathing became irregular and fast. The few seconds I spent in the red zone taught me one clear lesson about how color affected my body. And red was definitely not for me! Sliding to my right placed me in the cool, soothing shades of the blue-green end of the spectrum. Ah, that felt fantastic. My whole body seemed to drop its tensions, as the colors covered my entire face. My eyes felt relaxed and wide open. Normally I had to squint in bright light, but this was very different. It just felt good. Paying heed to the motto "If it feels good, do it," I did it.

Every day for a week, I rushed home and waited for the light show. I had to keep moving because the colors gradually slid into nothingness as the sun fell lower in the sky. Staying only in the blue-green district, with Ru sitting on my lap, I soaked in those rays and the time passed all too quickly. We both looked forward to our daily color time together.

⁕

Very early in life, Ru worked out the job description of what a mom should do and what a kid should do. It was a mom's job to cook, clean, and do just about everything. His job was to play—and he worked very hard at it.

Ru particularly loved playing outside our apartment, and on more than one occasion he came in for dinner after having left his toys all over the front yard. Not to worry, though. If he didn't bring his little treasures in, he had a mother to do it for him, right? It was in her job description.

Our building faced the street, and though the neighborhood was nice and safe, leaving toys out overnight—especially his tricycle—just was not prudent. That's why my toy-gathering duties sometimes took me and my virtually nonexistent night-vision out after dark.

Walking from our apartment to the front yard required going down three stairs, a nightmare for me, since the porch light didn't work. And I didn't have a flashlight. If Ru was already asleep, I usually wouldn't wake him just to help me pick up his toys. I must have been a sight to any neighbors looking out their window, as I crawled around on my hands and knees, using the touch-method to search for my child's abandoned toys. I especially disliked hitting something I wasn't expecting—like a snail or the results of a dog's defecation. Indeed, picking up Ru's toys after dark was an act of true motherly love.

One evening, I remembered well after dark that I needed to forage in the front yard for his neglected possessions. As I stepped out on the front porch, I realized immediately that I could see the three steps leading to the yard and, by some miracle, I could also see the toys on the grass. My initial reaction was to think the porch light had been fixed. One glance upward told me that was not the case.

Perhaps a brighter street light? No, at least not within my view. A full moon? No, the moon still hadn't made its appearance. What then?

My God, I was dumbfounded! The only thing I had been doing differently was sitting in the bath of color in the afternoons. Could that have had an effect? Could a color bath cause me to see better at night? Was such a completely strange thing possible?

Excitement overtook my senses. Hope was springing forth like a restless horse waiting to charge through the starting gate at the racetrack. My mind was moving a mile a minute. Had I somehow stumbled across a cure? I was thanking all my spiritual guides, the benevolent teachers along the way who have always been happy to share knowledge with me. I was grateful to my instincts for letting me act upon my desire to simply sit in the stream of color that my ten-gallon fish tank produced every afternoon.

But it seemed too simple. Too easy. No one was going to believe this. I had a lot of research to do. In order to really accept this simple answer, I decided I had to find out everything I could about color.

Could color be healing? I had never heard of such a thing and it certainly was odd. If I couldn't find some logical explanation, then my enthusiasm was probably all for nothing, and this was just some odd stage of my eye disease. A reprieve for the moment, not something that would last. Besides, how could I attribute my night vision improvement to color?

Finally, I calmed down enough to go to bed. Just as sleep embraced me, I wondered where to go to study color. I knew of no classes at the college. Who knew about color? The answer was simple—Collette! As an artist, she knew a great deal about it. Collette knew things like how to make complex colors out of simple, primary colors. As I drifted off to dreamland, I smiled gently to myself. I would call on Collette the very next day, after my classes.

She was home and very helpful. She had a book on the history of color called The Rainbow Book, with the individual chapters printed in different colors. I was astonished to read that the Egyptians, in 1500 B.C., used colors in their healing arts. When I realized their healers had even been sophisticated enough to perform brain surgery, I was intrigued. Reading further, I nearly dropped the book. I felt as if it had bitten me! The color that Egyptian healers used for treating eye disease was, of all things, blue-green! I was vindicated. I didn't know how, but everything began to make sense to me. I hadn't discovered something new; I had rediscovered something old.

As my quest for knowledge regarding color and light grew, I realized I needed to know even more about the eye disease I was fighting. If I hoped to develop a logical, orderly plan of action, I needed information. I had exhausted the data that the college anatomy lab had available on the eye.

In the early Seventies, much about how the eyes functioned was still a mystery. None of my technical questions were being answered to my satisfaction, at least here at the local level. Where else could I go? Upon asking the question, I immediately realized the answer. The University of California Medical Center in San Francisco.

After the original diagnosis of RP, the Medical Center was one place I had gone in search of other opinions. While nobody was able to help me, I did turn out to be helpful to them. I permitted the students to examine my eyes for practice at diagnosing RP. And what I now recalled was that once, while waiting for an examination to begin, I wandered through the many corridors there and stumbled upon the entrance to the medical library. That, I realized, would be an ideal place for me to start my investigation into the medical view of RP and other eye disorders. Without hesitation, I decided to journey to San Francisco on my next day off from college.

Getting to the Medical Center was complex. The bus from Santa Rosa took almost three hours, then I had to transfer three times on the San Francisco transit system. I once knew the Muni Bus system inside out, but now using it was not as easy, since I was out of practice getting around the city. Late in the afternoon, I finally found my way to the medical library. I wouldn't have much time for my search, as the time for me to return to Santa Rosa was near. I couldn't risk being out after dark. Knowing I would be lost without help, I began to get a little panicky.

The real kicker, I discovered, was that the library was closed to outsiders. You had to be a doctor or a student doctor or a member of the Medical Center staff. Not even a peek. The doors were closed, and without my having proper authorization, they would stay closed. My blood boiled with the injustice of it all. The secrets of science were being denied to me. It wasn't fair.

On the long journey home, I had a lot of time to ponder my predicament. My energy was depleted; the whole trip had been in vain. The only thing that carried me through the miles home was my anger at the injustices in the world. It was also what would provide the drive for me to solve the problem.

That evening, back in the safety of my apartment, with Ru asleep in my lap, I told my friend and neighbor Judy of the ill-fated adventure. Judy was a dental assistant and we had become close friends. She commiserated with me and said she wished she could do something to help.

Then as she was leaving, I suddenly realized that Judy could help me! She was still wearing her white lab coat, having come directly over to my place after work. It was the beginning of a great plan to get into that library.

I would borrow one of Judy's lab coats, which were identical to the white coats worn by the doctors and students at the UC Medical Center. With the additions of a few accessories, I could turn myself into a student.

The local toy store had a sale on the doctor-kits that children love to play with. The plastic stethoscope looked realistic and would fit nicely in a side pocket, sticking out, obvious to anyone's first glance. My name tag was easy and affordable via the local print shop. A pair of used nurse's shoes from the Salvation Army Thrift Store completed the outfit. I could have fooled my mother with this getup. I was ready to go back to the medical library, under cover and in full disguise. By hook or by crook, I was going to get in there and gather the secrets I knew it held about my eye disease.

The next time, reaching San Francisco didn't take anywhere near as long. Now I knew the routes and transferring to the local bus was easier. I was carrying my disguise in a book bag. The first available ladies' room would provide the opportunity to get into my costume. If Superman could change in a phone booth, so could I.

Shortly thereafter, I was a student nurse.

After checking to make sure my disguise was perfect, I took a breath and started toward the library door. My heart was pounding. I was unbelievably nervous. I wondered what the punishment might be if I were caught in the sacred library. Images of torture from the Inquisition came to mind. But surely they wouldn't lock me up for the mild form of subterfuge I was perpetrating, would they? (Likewise, neither would they lock up an eighteen-year-old girl for three years for stealing a lecherous man's car, would they?) Finally, I set my fears aside, as my need to know more about this disease overrode any personal concerns I had. I moved toward—and through—the door.

It was a piece of cake. If anyone noticed my entrance, I wasn't aware of it. No bells went off; there were no shouts from suspicious librarians hired to protect the secrets housed in the medical library. I felt as if I outsmarted them all, as though I put one over on the entire medical community.

My excitement was short-lived. Being inside a research library was very confusing, even overwhelming. This wasn't like a simple, easy-access college library. I saw piles of papers and bookshelves filled with thin little reports. I didn't know where to begin. So, as in most things, I asked questions of anyone who would listen. Impatiently, and I must say almost rudely, I was pointed in the direction of the eye research section.

It was amazing. The reports on eye diseases were written in a complex jargon I didn't understand at all. Not having been exposed to medical journals before, I realized I now must learn the code that doctors wrote in—complex language only other doctors could understand. I saw several books on the shelf that had multiple copies, found two with the most information on retinitis pigmentosa, and decided to take them home with me. I knew I'd need time to understand what they meant, and commuting every day would have been impossible. The only answer was to "borrow" them. That was all right. I'd bring them back. If anyone wanted those particular books before I returned, the remaining copies would meet their needs.

The search was discouraging at first, but with grim determination and a large magnifying glass in hand, I began the slow and laborious process of translating the terminology of investigative ophthalmology into simple English. Finally, after I'd gone through several sets of medical dictionaries and a few migraine headaches, I finished. Most of the difficult language was now understandable to me and I had a firm understanding of how a scientific paper gets written.

But my quest for answers brought up more questions. The medical community still did not fully understand the process involved in retinitis pigmentosa. Therefore, in their opinion, no treatment or cure existed. Until complete analysis was accomplished, no one would begin the search for a treatment—at least that's the impression I got. It was disheartening. However, since I had begun to notice improvement in my own visual function, I knew I must be doing something that affected the health of the eyes. In no way was that "all in my head" or part of a placebo effect.

The placebo effect. Apparently—I learned—in some trials of new drugs, two groups of people with the same medical problem are given samples of pills to take. One group (and which group is known only to the researchers) is given "sugar pills" and the other is given real medication. Some individuals in the group on the fake pills always report relief of symptoms. In other words, they believe the "medication" is going to help, and it does. That was the so-called "placebo effect." When I found out about it, I recognized how powerful the mind can be and wondered if my own improvement was due simply to my wanting to see better, if it was somehow less than real, perhaps impermanent, the result of a mental trick. However, my intuition told me my improved sight was based on actual, objective, physical improvement.

With the progress I was experiencing, I began to realize I had stumbled intuitively onto some alternative approaches to improving the sight in my eyes—perhaps in everyone's eyes. For example, in researching the nature of retinitis pigmentosa, I found that no one had ever reported improvement. A few cases reported an absence of change for a number of years, which was noteworthy, but no cases of out-and-out improvement were on record. Traditionally, the nature of the disease was that people lost about fifteen percent of their sight annually. Some would even lose much more in a shorter period of time. But there was no improvement. Except in my case. Dr. Jebrock's periodic tests showed actual increased visual function.

My relationship with Dr. Jebrock had matured into a strong friendship. Larry was always happy to see me, showing interest in my latest progress in research and experimentation. He, interestingly enough, had also been studying the effects of color on the visual system, so our sharing information was productive to us both. We made a great team and I asked Larry for a job working with him. I hoped to be able to give nutritional consultations and evaluations to people interested in improving their vision by changing their diet. Larry was interested in expanding his services and I began to work in his optometric office. We were definitely pioneering a new and exciting field—Holistic Optometry.

For me, it meant returning to Novato, a twenty-minute bus ride from Santa Rosa. And luck was with me. Ru and I moved in with Sylvia, a friend I met through college. We found a place just two blocks from Larry's office, a wonderful house with lots of windows and a big back yard. Life was going great. I was doing the work I truly wanted to do and, little by little, apparently getting better.

Sylvia was a trained masseuse, specializing in shiatsu, a form of acupressure more advanced than ordinary massage. Massage by itself is very helpful, especially in reducing muscle tension, which leads to increased circulation. However, with specialized training, Sylvia learned about the particular points on the body that, when activated, appeared to improve health even further. She was happy to share her knowledge with me. Further, working on the body was, for me, like finding a nice place to live: it felt good. Ru also benefited, since I did much work on him, often while he was asleep. Prevention continued to be uppermost in my mind for him.

⊙❧

Finally, the various approaches I was taking to improve my vision seemed all to come together, seemed all to be part of a larger pattern that could lead to visual wellness.

I saw confirmation in the outside world of some things I was doing to help my own vision improve. The medical community was beginning to accept the same general processes of visualization I used to increase the oxygen supply to my eyes. I even read a book—Getting Well Again by O. Carl Simonton and several co-authors—which described the successful use of guided visualization by terminally ill cancer patients, some of whom actually went into remission.

Official medical science, however, wasn't excited about the prospect of anyone's blending physical and mental therapies. The old belief system, ingrained for centuries, was hard to overcome. It was simple. Several hundred years before, Western philosophers had concluded that the body is mechanical, completely separate from and unaffected by the mind. The entire structure of modern medicine was based on those assumptions—regarded by most doctors as "facts."

Fortunately, many advanced thinkers are developing methods to better understand the relationship between thought and physical being, recognizing that the mind and body influence each other. I had often heard people say you can "worry yourself sick." Understanding that every story has at least two sides, I began to believe you could "think yourself well."

Balanced nutrition was an obvious contributor to well-being, although I hadn't been lucky enough to find a particular diet to make my eyes better. But eating a balanced diet had made my overall health much better.

The eye exercises were now part of a daily routine for Ru and me. Working with Larry gave me access to more-advanced color therapy instruments, as well as a better understanding of how they work. The mystery of color and light had begun to unravel under closer observation. Color is light, and light is vibration. Just as sound penetrates through one's system, so does light. The eyes are a natural for color therapy. They depend upon light stimulation in order to function. My intuition was right on the button the day I began to sit in my color bath.

Now, getting acupressure treatments from Sylvia, I began to see how the different approaches to well-being were all interconnected; all worked from different angles to give me the best vision I could possibly have. This wasn't a cure yet, but I felt I was on solid ground, developing a comprehensive and effective therapy plan. My disjointed journey on the way to better sight was becoming clearer. The road signs along the way were easy to identify.

⟨⟩

My family were wonderful volunteers for my new therapy. Mom was great, and whenever I found a new technique to be helpful, she came down for dinner and a treatment. She was a willing, intelligent guinea pig. Ru was okay, but couldn't really give me the adult feedback I needed to evaluate the therapy further. The only time Ru was not willing was when I began studying acupuncture. He, at the very precious age of five, refused to let me practice my needlework on him. Nothing I did or said could convince him to get up on the massage table. Arms folded across his chest, lower lip stubbornly stuck out, he refused to budge.

"But Ru, who can I practice on?" I asked, trying to get him to give in. Ru calmly looked around for an alternative and spotted our old dog, Jake.

"Do him," he commanded, pleased to have come up with an answer so fast. He was quick that day. Living with me was honing his survival skills.

Faithful old Jake, not all that willingly, became a pin cushion to practice on. All I can say is that until the day Jake died, he had more energy and spark, and never seemed to be bothered by the arthritis that had been settling in his back legs. It didn't happen on the first treatment, but over a period of a month, he was definitely better.

Jake notwithstanding, Ru still wasn't willing. He had drawn his line in the sand, and I admired his grit.

I had to give up acupuncture because I could never have passed the test in California. It was the first state to exact laws allowing people to practice acupuncture and the examination was among the most difficult anywhere. To qualify, I would have been asked to identify capillaries on a test subject, and I couldn't have done it. However, the knowledge I gained from studying acupuncture was invaluable. It was powerful, and it gave me a totally different approach to thinking of illness and disease. I hadn't wasted the time.

10

ROAD SIGNS

Rain had fallen all morning. I was due in the office at one in the afternoon.

Collette dropped by for a visit and touching base with her was good because we hadn't seen one another in a while. She and I had gone through fire together and our friendship was solid. But she was a bad girl this afternoon. Collette wanted company for a trip to the beach. As an artist, she liked the stormy days, claiming they inspired her more than the boring, sunny days there. I had to agree with her about that. Storms would whip the surf into a frenzy, and it was exciting.

I wanted to go, but had to work. Collette looked sad for me. I decided to give in. The office wasn't too happy about my late cancellation, but this was one of the first times I ever missed work. To justify such behavior, I checked this off as a mental health day.

Massive rain clouds covered the countryside as we headed to the beach. On the way, driving along the two-lane curved country road with hills on either side, Collette looked in her rearview mirror and stopped the car immediately.

"Look at the rainbows," she sputtered excitedly to me. My initial reaction was not to look, since seeing rainbows was normally impossible for me. Usually I looked in the direction others were looking as they admired the art show of the sky, but I couldn't see it.

To humor Collette, I looked in the general direction she indicated. Amazingly, I was able to see it—the most gorgeous sight I had ever seen. In a valley with beautifully sculpted green hills, I saw two rainbows, end to end. Their colors were so vivid! I had never seen two rainbows like that, nor did I even know they could exist. It was, I decided, a magic show that God puts on only once in a while. The best part, of course, was that I could see them, truly see them. Collette and I just stood there hugging one another. She was aware what a personal achievement it was for me to see any rainbow at all, but this one was really special. I took it as a sign that I was on the right road to fully recovering my sight.

We headed for a remote beach called Limontour. It is a favorite of mine, a long stretch of white beach with hills on one end that stretch out to the Pacific Ocean. The water was motley greys and blues; dark, puffy rain clouds scattered above cast giant shadows. We sat on top of a sand dune to get a good look at the sea.

When I looked up, I almost fainted. It was as if the earth beneath me started spinning. I automatically reached out to touch something, to balance my body. The shock of what I was witnessing was too great.

Normally when I went to the beach, seeing things was like looking through a tunnel. I could see the sand, if I was looking right at it. If I turned to look at the ocean, I could not see the sand. If I turned to look at the sky, I could not see the sand, nor the blue ocean. My vision was so narrow that panoramic views were impossible for me to take in. I had to do it piecemeal, one view at a time.

On this magical day, when I looked up and out, I saw the sky, the water, the sand, and even the cliffs at the end of the beach. For the first time, I was able to see the whole picture! It was almost too much for me to take. I was in shock, unable to understand what was happening. Only with Collette's gentle assistance was I able to finally grasp the significance of what was going on. All the work I had done, the therapies I gradually included, had allowed my sight to become the best I'd ever had as an adult! This indeed was a special day. The twin rainbows were only the beginning.

Collette and I talked on the way back to Novato. I told her I must now go to the medical community to show them I was better. Maybe they could help other people save their sight as well. It was a difficult decision since I had been put off by the attitudes of the eye specialists I dealt with in the past. But I knew it had to be done. I couldn't keep this a secret, helping only my family and myself. Too many people in the world were suffering daily from loss of sight and I wanted to share what I'd just found out about my own improvement. In my heart, I knew the medical establishment would be happy to help the people they turned away before, the people to whom they offered no hope. Of course, there was hope. Without hope, our lives are empty shells, and we're waiting for the end to come in order for the spirit to move on—and that's for those lucky enough to believe in the spirit. For the others, it's really bleak.

The next morning I called my retinal specialist in San Francisco. We set an appointment for the end of the week. He was one of the most sought-after specialists in the United States and had been interested in my retinas because I had some unusual qualities he wanted to include in his forthcoming book. I had gone through the required tests, one of which—the electroretinogram—had been terribly painful. It is considered an objective test, since the physiological function of the retina can be measured without verbal input from the patient. Subjective tests, not considered reliable by medical researchers, are those in which the patient has to answer questions, interpreting or acknowledging what's going on.

The last time I had taken the electroretinogram, the doctors said I would never have to take it again. That didn't upset me, until I asked them why not. It was a bittersweet predicament. The test showed I had a "flat line"—my retinas were shot, not responding to light. In other words, I had a major problem and it wasn't going to get better. The reason I wasn't ever going to have to take the test again was that, in their view, no one recovers from a flat line. Until now, that is!

My doctor was surprised when I asked to be referred to the hospital for another electroretinogram. I told him I wanted to take it again, and after the results were evaluated, I would tell him my reasons. I didn't want to tell him beforehand, as it might have altered his decision to let me get another examination. Besides, he owed me for all the times I let him take pictures of the back of my eyes for his book. Quid pro quo.

Returning to the same room, to the same machine, I submitted my eyes to this torture test. After about ten drops of dilation fluid are put in, drops that sting like acid but numb the eyeball, a huge contact lens is put in each eye. It's called a sclera contact lens, covering the white of the eyes, thus keeping the lids wide and painfully open. Tiny electrodes are attached to the outside of the contact lens. Get the picture? It sounds like something out of the terrifying science fiction movie A Clockwork Orange, doesn't it? It was not pleasant.

After the technician hooked me up, I was left alone in the dark for twenty minutes. With eyes forced to stay open by oversized contact lenses, all I could do was relax, or try to relax. As I lay on the uncomfortable table, I began to expand my awareness, breathing deeply, letting go of all tension and fear. I tried to see what I could in this dark, windowless room. My memory of the previous test was that I couldn't see a thing; the room took on overtones of a tomb or a cave. Now, as I lay in the same darkness, I began to notice little sources of light. The button on the telephone on the desk was blinking. I could see it! From the glow the button produced, I was able to make out the outline of the phone itself. That had not been possible on my last visit.

With an overwhelming sense of confidence and peace, I waited for the test to begin. I knew, without a doubt, that my vision was better and that the improvement would show up on this particular test. Knowing is half the battle.

The technician began to run the test. After getting accustomed to the dark, the assistant would start flashing extremely bright strobe lights directly above my eyes, eyes that couldn't protect themselves against the vicious and blinding onslaught. The strobe started slow, building up at different stages of the test to a blinking rate that would irritate a disco dancer. The exam didn't take long once they began the light show. The electrodes recorded the ability of my retinas to process light. The last test score had been a big zero, the "flat line."

After I got the contacts out of my eyes, my lids began to blink, trying to catch up with what they had been missing for nearly an hour. Although my pupils were the size of grapes, I was happy. An inner part of my being knew I had done well. The pain and agony were worth it if the evidence backed up my claim of improvement. Then, with the interest and support of the medical community, I could begin to help others. After all, that was why I put myself through this agony.

Collette and I waited in the lobby until the doctor came to discuss the results. This was a doctor I had not seen before, and he was unaware that I had exposed myself to this kind of eye exam a few years earlier. I wanted it that way so he was not prejudiced, and would give me his fresh opinion.

His face was solemn as he walked toward our corner. In his hands, he carried the long strip of paper that would tell the tale.

"Miss Halloran," he said sadly, "the results show that you have some peaks, but your response was in the low-normal range." As I looked at the ticker-type tape, even I could see the lines that jumped up and down all the way through the test. Collette and I started hugging each other with contagious joy. The doctor was totally confused.

"I don't think you understand what this means, Miss Halloran." He tried to inject a more sober tone into our celebration. "It means your eyes aren't normal, and your probably have some visual dysfunction due to the lack of normal response." He was trying his best to let me know what the results meant to him.

It was time to let him in on my secret. When I told him I was there only a few years ago and had been shown to have a flat line, he looked incredulous. "How can that be?" he asked, shaking his head as if to clear his brain of cobwebs. In all fairness, I have to recognize that he tried to hold onto his professional demeanor. But it was falling apart. He had never heard of anyone's electroretinogram getting better.

I didn't need to explain to him. I did need to talk to my own doctor and quickly, about this exciting evidence of improvement. I knew he was in for a big surprise. I was so happy, I couldn't stop grinning. Collette was just as happy for me.

I returned to my regular doctor with the evidence in black and white. He began a thorough examination of the back of my eyes. The exam light shining into my eyes seemed almost pale in comparison to the harsh lights I experienced earlier. My eyes were still dilated, so his close inspection was easy.

He was making small sounds as he looked closer. Sounds like humm humm that became higher and higher with each humm he uttered, as if in surprise and disbelief.

"What do you see?" I asked impatiently.

He wouldn't tell me until he started to write down his observations. Thumbing through his records of my past visits, he started shaking his head.

"I wish I had made...an exact record of the pigmentation pattern, because even though I will deny it in public, it seems that you have less pigment discoloration than you did on previous visits." He couldn't be sure, but I knew he was right. I think he knew he was right, too. He just wouldn't go out on a limb without hard evidence to back up his claim. He was caught in the quandary of medical science's rules and regulations. Besides, he was the President of the Northern California Ophthalmological Society. He was a bigwig in as established and conservative order and couldn't risk his reputation. He admitted it to me almost apologetically. At least he had the guts to tell me the truth.

"What I can do is write a letter of introduction to a doctor I know who is doing research on RP," he said. A researcher who could determine whether, in fact, I had improved from a traditionally degenerative eye disease. Willing and read to go to the scientists, I accepted his offer.

Collette and I celebrated all over two counties on our way home. She was my best friend and knew how important the results were. She was also excited about my upcoming meeting with the Research Scientist. Getting the appointment would take a couple of weeks, but I wasn't worried. I knew my visual improvement wasn't temporary. It would wait for further investigation.

As the meeting day approached, my friends and coworkers were supportive and excited. Larry Jebrock helped me gather my visual field test records, showing the expansion over the few years we had worked together. Those records, combined with my visual acuity improvement, detailed my progress. The tests Larry compiled were subjective, since I had to give input. But the electroretinogram was the icing on the cake. Its results, its objective results, verified the other measurements. I knew I had a strong case to present.

⟨❧⟩

In spite of my confidence, I was nervous while I waited in the Research Scientist's office, in a part of the Medical Center in San Francisco that was unfamiliar to me. But I wasn't nervous about talking with him. I was nervous about the little tingle in my conscience when I remembered I'd never returned the research books I borrowed from the Medical Library several years earlier.

Our appointment was scheduled for ten o'clock in the morning. Ten forty-five was fast approaching. Even research scientists keep you waiting. Maybe it's something they learn in school. Like, get a good tax lawyer and CPA, wear white, drive a foreign car, a sports car if you're single, a sedan if you're married, and, last but not least, keep your patients waiting. These rules seem to be along the same lines as learning to write so no one else can read it. Same principle, I'm sure.

This doctor, the first real scientist I'd come across, showed up nearly fifty minutes late. Barely looking at me, then glancing at his digital watch, he said he could only give me ten minutes. He said he had an important experiment due in a few minutes and would be leaving soon. Nice opening, I thought.

Okay, I said to myself, this doctor really doesn't want to be here with me. I took a deep breath and began my story of hard work and positive results. I had rehearsed what I was going to say. My coworkers at the office showed me how to give a brief, intelligent, and semi-scientific presentation. No emotions, they warned; no words like terrific or fabulous. Words like ERG, Snellen Acuity, Ishihara Color Examination. These were the buzzwords to use when talking to a scientist involved with eye research. Just the facts. But I could tell he was getting interested. He sat down, moving off the corner of his desk. He leafed through the papers I laid out, which—in chronological order—backed up each claim I made.

"How and what do you think caused these test results?" he asked. I noticed he didn't use the word "improvement." I began to tell him about my nutritional changes, the supplements I took, my eye exercises, and the techniques for stress management and visualization. I left nothing out, describing my daily routine for stronger and healthier eyes.

That he was shaking his head slowly from side to side clued me to the possibility of his not accepting my explanation. It was clear I had lost him when I gave more than one factor for the possible change in my test results. He was a "one cause, one effect" kind of guy.

As swiftly as a surgeon cuts into a patient, this doctor started to take me apart. A bedside manner isn't usually required if one works with lab rats. He was cruel with his words, certainly not caring I was in the room.

He began with the result of the recent electroretinogram. The batteries could have been different, the technician was new. In other words, the parameters of the test were not exact. Even though it was the same hospital and the same machine, there were differences any true scientist could shoot holes through. Second, my test results proved nothing. This was not a scientific presentation. Laboratory controls had not been established. He was intent in naming off the reasons why my improvement was not properly documented. Instead of really hearing what I was saying, that indeed I did see better, he was criticizing my methods. His background and training didn't allow him to listen. His belief was that this disease had no cure, no treatment. Anyone who said otherwise was incorrect.

Early in my discourse, I established that my friends and associates and I were not scientists. We had gathered as much data as possible, hoping a scientific study would come out of this meeting. Although I did not say to him in so many words, I wasn't here to get his approval or acceptance of the evidence I had collected. Our hope was to get his interest and then his help in setting up a valid, acceptable study of the methods and the results.

He wasn't interested. He told me that when I had collected several hundred test results from other patients, and when he could duplicate the results in his laboratory, then and only then would we have something. Until that happened, he told me, I was wasting his time.

In a fit of anger and frustration, I retorted, "Fine, when you reach the point where you and your rats can communicate, I will be happy to come back and show you how to get these results!" He looked surprised at my outburst, then uncomfortable. With a wave of his hand, as if to dismiss my accusation, he was out of the door.

I went down like a hot-air balloon that suddenly has a large hole in it. My confidence was gone, and the only thing left for me to do was to cry. So that's what I did, most of the way home. My first meeting with a scientist had been a disaster. Now what was I to do? All my dreams of being able to help others and to get a real, close, scientific study of my program were shot to pieces.

Walking up the drive to my house, I noticed a few more cars than usual around the street. I had forgotten that some of my friends would come over to help celebrate and to find out what happened in my meeting with "Mr. Wizard."

Their cheers of welcome were short-lived as they noticed the sad face I was wearing. Ru rushed over to give me a hug, and I held on to him fiercely as I started relating my tale of complete failure. Larry and Ellen had come over after work. Without their words of comfort and encouragement, I don't think I ever would have tried again.

They weren't surprised at the doctor's reaction. Scientists are a unique breed of humans, Larry told us later. They don't hear what you're saying, and they need to prove everything to themselves, often in rigid and unyielding ways. Remember, he said, they still believe the body and mind are two separate entities, not aspects of a whole, as we have come to realize.

I felt better, and my spirits began to rise. That rejection was the first real wall I had come up against, and I almost collapsed. Thank God for my friends. Without their support, I might have bounced back, but I don't think it would have happened as soon as the next day.

If I needed more evidence, then, by God, I would amass tons of it. I knew the program worked. My mother knew it and had begun to benefit from doing the work. My little boy had eagle eyes and was often my guide. I didn't need the approval of a Man of Science. At least, not now. If doing so took years, I was determined to prove the program worthy of a closer look. That was only logical. In the meantime, at least we were all enjoying the benefits of improved sight. Just because a scientist wouldn't study the program didn't meant we weren't getting results. I didn't need his approval to know I was seeing better.

My own sight was my scientific proof. But I had learned my lesson well. If I were to help other people with serious eye disorders, I had to get the medical community to look at the results and at the program itself. Without a double blind study (excuse the pun), including a report published in an approved medical journal, I wouldn't be of any real help to anyone. Only with those things done would the program I had developed be accepted. Doing all that would be hard and would take time, but I was willing to do it. My confidence was reborn. With supportive friends and family, I began to formulate a plan of attack.

Dr. Jebrock, my friend and employer, was open to suggestions. I said I wanted to begin spreading the word that we had a program for people with RP. With his help and his evaluations, we could begin collecting the documentation needed to convince the scientific community.

Within a few days, a friend was able to get me interviewed by our local newspaper. The Independent Journal was a county-wide newspaper, a daily, well-read and well-respected. The first article about my work appeared on January 8, 1976, my daughter's eighth birthday. It was quite a day to celebrate, though my cheer was dampened by the reopening of that wound of the heart. I missed my daughter still.

Intuitively, I felt she was living in Marin County. The night my article came out, I lay awake for hours, thinking about her. How was she? Was she healthy? Maybe her parents had received the Independent Journal that very day. Somehow I knew I had to leave large footprints for her to follow.

I was certain we would be together again, someday. That the first article had been in a Marin newspaper was, I felt, a good omen. I was determined to make a name for myself, one that would be visible, to guide my daughter's search.

I was told many times that after an adopted child turns eighteen, she can have access to her adoption records, if she desires. I knew she would come looking for me. I wanted to make finding me easy.

I told Ru again about his sister the next morning, and he was excited. He wanted her to come looking for us right then. I explained to him that she was still too young, that we would have to wait at least ten more years. Ru said okay, but he would be all grown up, too. As we hugged each other, I could feel my heart start to heal once again. My son's young, healthy arms gave me such love, and that helped ease the pain.

⊙❧

The newspaper story was very favorable and the response was tremendous. The phone at Larry's office was busy for several weeks after the article came out. People were intrigued by the fact that one of their own, a fellow RP sufferer, had beaten the odds, had actually gone against the grain of the usual prognosis. Before long, people other than my family were trying my program and working with Dr. Jebrock.

We were on the path to sharing our success. After all, I didn't want my family to be the only ones benefiting from this. I wanted others to receive the same improvement we had. Now I just had to learn how to provide the information in a way that didn't take the five years I spent stumbling around looking here and there for answers. If the program were to be of any real benefit, it should have two important attributes. It should be easy to teach people, and its results should become evident within a few months.

My days were full and challenging. Many people with different eye problems wanted to be helped. I spent lots of nights involved with studies, evaluations, and a great deal of worry that the program wouldn't work on others. Doubts were always with me at night. During the day, I had confidence and a professional attitude I learned from Larry and Ellen. They were always calm and collected. I mimicked their stance and got away with it. Until I was alone at night, that is. From one side of midnight to the other, I pondered the program and the people I was working on. If I didn't get the worry under control, I knew stress would take its toll on my eyes. I needed to talk to someone about it all. But who?

Larry's reputation as an innovative and progressive optometrist had spread far. We even took on our first graduate of optometry college, in a training position. His name was Elliot Kaplan, and he was from the Boston area. He was young, attractive, and had the wonderful accent that travels with anyone from the East Coast. His enthusiasm was contagious, and we got along very well.

I felt that his understanding of eye problems from the patient's viewpoint was important. His interest was sincere. Together we ventured into the countryside on the weekends, and he always asked what I saw and how I viewed it. Then he compared my view to his own.

Within four walls, visual functions and testing are very limiting. The true test of vision is how one operates in the real world. Bright sunlight, shadows from the trees and buildings and mountains, and twilight time are among the possible configurations that affect the ability to see. Elliot was willing to explore these things, and he was schooled in the complex nature of sight. We became good friends, a friendship that has lasted well over fifteen years.

Elliot became the confidant and counselor I needed in matters concerning my eye program. Of special value to me was the fact that I was able to let him know my fears, so we could examine them together. There were times when I had little daydreams of Elliot and me working side-by-side, not only as colleagues but also as lovers. That never happened, but not because I hadn't thought about it.

The time came for another visual field test at the office. I was looking forward to this repeat because last time, although my vision had improved significantly, I was still legally blind. But just barely so. With only the slightest additional improvement I would enter the world of the legally sighted.

Elliot and Larry were both excited about my progressively improving visual field tests. Each of them had volunteered to give the forthcoming exam. Their attention and excitement made me feel like a giddy schoolgirl.

The night had been a good one for sleeping and my worries were on hold. Besides, I was getting fantastic feedback from my colleagues at work.

That was building my self-confidence and making my doubts seem like silly, neurotic worries.

That morning, as with every morning, I awoke and looked out my window to see what I could see. That day, as with every day, I thanked the heavens and my luck for seeing anything at all. Then, that day, I carefully evaluated what I saw, checking to determine whether anything was different. The leaves on the tree out back seemed to be more distinctive. I could see them individually, instead of the greenish blur that had been my only clue the leaves were still on the tree at all. I reveled in the different shades of green I could now distinguish. The warm brown and almost black tones of the branches and trunk were downright sensuous. No wonder I wanted to hug a tree. Excitedly, I prepared for work. My quarterly eye exam was on the slate for today.

We were using an old-fashioned but very effective field-of-vision test called a stereo-campimeter. I placed my chin in a cup and looked through a pair of binocular-type lenses. One was covered. A light was affixed to the top of the instrument, providing good and repeatable illumination. The distance, the lighting, and the size of the target were standardized, making the test very accurate.

The paper on which the test was recorded was a dull black, with faint white concentric circles, beginning with a small central circle and enlarging out to the edges, with the circles progressively ten degrees larger. A small X marked the center, where I would keep my eye focused. Dr. Jebrock slowly brought in a small white circular target on the end of a black felt wand. When the white target entered my field of sight, I acknowledged its presence out loud. The wand, being black felt, did not make a noise when it slid on the paper; it might come toward the center from any angle, without warning. If one couldn't see it until it got very close to or on the white X, then one's field of vision was significantly blocked. I knew that because, during my early years of getting examined, the target had to be almost right on the X for me to see it.

My emotions were at a fever pitch. I was blinking rapidly, and backed away from the instrument for a moment, wanting to collect myself. Letting go of any expectations, taking a deep breath, calming myself down, and relaxing as deeply as I could, I engaged the instrument again. Adjusting my eye to look at the X, I told Larry and Elliot I was ready to begin.

Then the most amazing thing happened. Without taking my eye off the middle target, the white X, I was able to see the white circular target off the side as it was first beginning to make its way towards the center. They mistook my scream for some kind of pain, rather than shock at seeing the circle target so quickly. Both Elliot and Larry must have jumped several feet in the air.

"I can see the target now!" I yelled, wanting them to understand the significance of what just happened.

"Try it again, Grace," Elliot said calmly, though I knew he was really excited.

Again, the same thing. I could see the target clearly, and as I studied the paper, I saw almost the entire page, even with its faint little white circles, all the way to the four corners. It was one of the most overwhelming moments of my life. My abdomen was tensing up as if to ward off a blow and I could hardly breathe. This was far more than I expected, more than I dared to dream. The central field of vision in my left eye was almost normal—an unbelievable accomplishment, considering that two years earlier I was supposed to be totally blind.

The office was in total chaos with excitement and joy. I tested equally well with my other eye. All the patients in the waiting room were smiling nervously. They were happy, but didn't understand the significance of the event. On the other hand, Larry, Elliot, and Ellen could barely maintain their professional demeanor for the rest of the day. We were making history. My experience at the beach had been validated by this test, and it was truly exhilarating. My feet didn't touch the ground all day.

Only after I got into bed did the reality begin to sink in. This meant only one thing. I could get a car! The test would qualify me for a driver's license, and that meant mobility and freedom!

Life was good. Now I could sleep knowing that what I had discovered wouldn't help just me, but would prevent my child from suffering the loss the medical establishment had predicted. I slept the sound sleep of someone with nothing to worry about. I began to dream about the kind of car I was going to get. Would it be a sporty number? A practical station wagon? What? The issue became one of identity. What kind of person was I? It seems one is what one drives, not what one eats. As I slid deeper into sleep, I felt a small smile playing on my lips. It didn't matter what I would drive, even it if was a tank. The fact was, I could drive now.

11

NOW I SEE

Our beautiful little pickup truck was a brilliant, fire-engine-red, rotary-engine Mazda. It had a stereo and tape player with terrific speakers. Ru was thrilled. It seemed made to order for us. Especially since I initially thought it was a four-wheel drive truck. (Yes, I should have checked it out better, but I just didn't know that much about trucks.) Tossing sleeping bags and barbecue equipment into the back made our outings freewheeling, spur-of-the-moment, and inexpensive. Ru's twin bed mattress fit perfectly in the rear. Our weekends were going to be different from now on. We would hit the road Friday afternoon and return late Sunday.

No one ever appreciated the outdoors and the highways as I did. They were a gift. Now, with the return of mobility, my feelings of appreciation and gratitude brought tears of joy to my eyes. People must have thought we were a tad backwards, singing and laughing as we traveled the byways and back roads into the wilderness. Often I turned the truck onto a dirt trail, off the paved road, to find a secluded part of the redwood forest. Had I known I didn't have four-wheel drive capability at the beginning, I'm sure it all wouldn't have been as much fun.

Finding a quiet spot when the sunset was long past, Ru and I got into the back of the truck, fluffed up our pillows, and snuggled into our sleeping bags. We told each other stories and enjoyed one another's company in the quiet woods.

Waking up to sunlight filtering through the cathedral ceiling of treetops was breathtaking, almost a religious experience. The silence was profound, and Ru and I gently eased ourselves to a sitting position, watching carefully for the shy forest dwellers. We would see the mamma deer with their babies, nibbling away at the emerald green grass that carpeted the forest floor. Squirrels chattered away to one another, discussing which little tidbit to save or devour. I was sure we would see Thumper any moment, trailing behind his friend Bambi.

This was what having a vehicle meant to me—the luxury of getting out into the countryside, to breathe in the smells of earth, damp with the morning dew. I hadn't realized how much I missed it until I was able to have the experience again.

⁂

My little boy was growing up, developing his own personality. It wasn't uncommon for people to tell me how handsome he was and that he had the most beautiful eyes they had ever seen. My heart would swell with pride, as if I could take credit for his good looks. Every night while he slept, I gently massaged his acupressure points, stimulating the energy pathways that would keep his vision strong. Doing eye exercises was still part of our daily routine. Neither of us had tired of the discipline. Besides, thanks to that discipline—thanks to determination and persistence—we were now travelling around in our own red truck. The lessons of earning our rewards were well understood by us both. We'd be registering no complaints when we got results like these. Every day was one of surprise, full of visual treats. Sunsets and sunrises were etched in my memory, with colors and beauty that could not have been appreciated more by the greatest artists or photographers. The temptation to stop and look at everything and anything was often too great. Giving in to that temptation just brought me more pleasure.

❧

As all of this was going on, thoughts of my daughter popped up at the oddest times. I would see a young girl at the shopping center and wonder: is she my child?

After the article about my success was published on her birthday, I decided to write the Marin Adoption Agency. I wanted to tell them of the discovery of the eye problem in my family, since it could be important to my daughter's medical history. I delayed because I didn't want to send information to the adoptive parents that was negative and without hope. Now, with my sight improved and a program in its infancy to help others, I felt the time had arrived to share this with the adoption agency. I hoped they would pass the information along to her parents.

The programming had been thorough at the time I signed the adoption papers. They made it clear to me in no uncertain terms that I would not have access to any information regarding my child. By signing the papers, I gave up any right to know of her life. So my letter was brief, and it took every ounce of courage I had not to ask how she was, where she lived, and whether she was safe and happy. I did send a copy of the newspaper article and a brief history of the eye disease, but I never heard from the adoption agency or the parents. All I could do was hope the message had been passed along.

⊘≫

Living in Marin County, north of San Francisco, during the Seventies provided unique educational opportunities. Marin had become the birthplace for and mecca of holistic medicine and holistic health care in the United States. My working at Dr. Jebrock's office provided me with many benefits, including introductions to new and exciting alternative healing methods. New opportunities appeared on a daily basis, for the network of holistic practitioners was one of the largest in the country.

I was invited to lecture at the Wholistic Health and Nutrition Institute (WHN) in Mill Valley, where they were establishing one of the first Natural Healing Colleges. Amazingly, I was able to be a teacher and a student at the same time. My field-of-vision therapy utilizing natural methods was unique and my skills and knowledge were welcomed. In exchange, I was able to attend many classes they offered. My education was expanding and my views about health opened up to new ideas. Ironically, some of those "new" ideas were over six thousand years old, as they were based on ancient Oriental principles of health and healing. Blending Oriental philosophy with the New Age health therapies was a natural.

The people I met, most of whom were involved with the healing arts, were genuine and caring. There were doctors, nurses, and other health professionals with conventional medical backgrounds. Usually they were burnt-out on the traditional approach of using allopathic medication—drugs—for most of their patients' complaints. The more medication they prescribed, the sicker their patients often became. As caring individuals, they sought alternative forms of therapy, ones that did not create more problems.

After almost six months of attending classes and teaching, I was asked to become part of the clinical staff at Wholistic Health and Nutrition. The director, a bona fide medical doctor, suggested that I head up a Wholistic Vision Clinic at the center. It was a wonderful opportunity. However, it meant leaving Larry Jebrock's office.

Because Larry had been my mentor for almost five years and a good friend, my decision was difficult, but he was understanding and encouraged me to branch out. The change made sense, especially if I was going to specialize in working with people who had serious eye disorders. Larry's main thrust, by contrast, was dealing with clients who wanted alternatives to wearing glasses, and people who availed themselves of his specialized vision training and therapy were either myopic or farsighted.

Within two months, I was a full-time teacher and staff member at WHN, which was a ten-minute drive north of the Golden Gate Bridge. Ru and I stayed in Novato, as I didn't want to take him out of school. Now that I was able to drive, the twenty-minute commute was a pleasure. When traffic was bumper-to-bumper, I smiled. "Well, you asked for it," I told myself, "and now you've got it. If you want to drive, expect delays along the way."

WHN was unique. Among the staff were medical doctors, nurses, practitioners, chiropractors, herbologists, acupuncturists, iridologists (who diagnose health problems by looking at the eye's iris), massage practitioners (including Rolfers), and me. The schedule was hectic. Each workday we gathered in the conference room for lunch to discuss cases we were working on. The interdisciplinary communication was educational and enlightening. If one of us had a difficult case, we presented a thorough medical history, then got feedback and questions from several different perspectives. Often one practitioner would spot an area that had been overlooked by another practitioner, and be able to offer a possible solution. I thought: if only traditional medicine could be guided into taking a more holistic approach.

Our clients were happy and successful for the most part. We all loved what we were doing, and by working together and assisting one another, we were unbeatable. It was a very exciting time for me and I loved the opportunity to learn about other health problems and their treatments. In my mind, I always applied the information to how it might affect the eyesight. It was a time of intense learning, an advanced course in alternative health services. And applying theory to practice was easy, since the Vision Clinic was beginning to gain recognition and I had people to work with.

Elliot Kaplan had left Larry's office to start his own practice, but he and I remained friends. The three of us, in fact, though going in our separate directions, all had shared special times together which would keep us friends for many years to come. Elliot was great. I found his sense of humor and his willingness to explore inner feelings to be wonderful qualities. It continued to be unrequited love on my side. Still, a woman could have her fantasies, right?

⬥

Marin County is an extremely wealthy locale. Prices were high, but the fascinating, wholeness-oriented lifestyle was worth it, and evoked envy from most people who visited the area. It wasn't uncommon to go to a friend's house for dinner and end up sipping sparkling apple cider in a hot tub for dessert. There's something about being naked together in bubbling hot water that brings people closer together. It is also very relaxing. Removing stress from the mind and the body became a passion of many people in Marin, and to a degree unsurpassed by any other group of people I'd heard of. Marin took on the look and feel of a very clean, semi-boiled, laid-back society, still dealing with the dog-eat-dog drive to get ahead, but in a very low-stress way.

The Marin County Fair was held around the Fourth of July. It was the best such event I ever attended. One low price got you in the Fair, which was spread over at least ten acres. Gourmet fast foods, handcrafted clothes, jewelry, and art were plentiful. The sun shone and the temperature soared up to at least ninety degrees during the day. Wonderful blue and white striped tents provided little islands of shade. The amusement rides, the best as far as I'm concerned, were the kind that travel from fair to fair.

All the rides were included in the price of admission, and I loved the scary ones. Ru and I would line up for the Hammer, the Octopus, the Zipper, and all the others that moved me to prayer. As soon as the ride began, I clung onto the protection bar with an iron grip.

That's when I communicated with God. "Please God," I said to myself, "just let me live through this ride and I promise, I'll never get on another one." Well, God learned not to trust me because the moment the ride slowed to a full stop, unlocked, and let us go free, I ran with Ru to get in line for the next scary one. What can I say? I must be a thrill seeker.

Riding the genuinely crazy rides gave me the opportunity to practice what I had learned about stress-management techniques and mental control. Relaxing under those extremely stressful circumstances was quite a challenge. But I got so good at it that I didn't have to hold the restraining bar. I became "one" with the twists and turns the machine took. It was an excellent place to practice the art of "letting go."

Many people were giving demonstrations of products or services. Chiropractors with their massage tables tested passersby to see if they were out of alignment, which was one way to educate the public and get new clients at the same time. Foot massagers were rubbing tired and sweaty feet for a dollar. Business cards, flyers, and leaflets littered the grounds like confetti after a New Year's Eve party.

One of the men demonstrating an unfamiliar body therapy caught my attention. He was standing next to a tall massage table. A gentleman was on the table, lying on his back. The man who was standing appeared to be moving or manipulating the other man's arms and legs, moving them up and down, sometimes sideways. It was intriguing, so I moved closer. Apparently, he was testing the strength in the man's muscles. Why was I suddenly interested, waiting for them to finish so I could ask questions? I didn't know.

After he was through, the man who had been lying down left the table, shaking his head as though in disbelief. It was obvious, even from where I stood, that something of benefit had happened to him. My curiosity got the better of me, making me impatient.

Then a young boy about my son's age came up to the demonstrator. I observed him closely, thinking this must be the man's son. He looked somehow different, not quite normal, but I couldn't identify at the moment what the difference was. He was obviously excited about being at the Fair, and from the way his father dug into his pocket, I'm sure the boy asked for more money. The process was familiar to me because my pockets were emptied several times during the day by identical requests. "More money, Mom," was the name I answered to, especially if games were nearby to be played.

After the man's son skipped happily off toward the amusements area, I was able to get close enough to start with my list of questions. First, though, to break the ice, I said I noticed his son was having a good time.

The look the father gave me was strange. I thought I saw the sparkle of a tear, though he immediately grinned from ear to ear, the way proud parents do when someone, anyone, mentions their children. I took a chance and asked why the tears, hoping his son wasn't ill.

The father, who introduced himself as Bill, told a most incredible story. Apparently his son, only two years prior to this very day, had been so severely mentally retarded that doctors recommended he be sent to an institution. He was not able to clothe himself or tie his shoes, and could barely feed himself. Then Bill came across the process he demonstrated to the man on the massage table. Created by Dr. John Thie, a chiropractor from Pasadena, California, it was called "Touch for Health." Bill learned it and applied its techniques every day for two full years on his son. The results, as I had seen in the earlier interaction, were little short of miraculous. They set my mind spinning.

If this technique could help his severely retarded son become nearly normal, what could it do for RP and eye diseases? I had to learn it. I asked Bill how and where I could get training in Touch for Health.

My intuition was working overtime. This, I knew, was a very important meeting, and not by accident did I start paying attention to what was going on at this corner of the Fair. My instincts took hold of my body and directed me to the demonstration area. Again, Something was guiding me to the right place at the right time. Quickly giving thanks to the Universe, I jotted down Bill's phone number and address, noting that he was giving an introductory workshop the next weekend. I made a mental note to be there, with bells on.

With that important meeting out of the way, I caught up with Ru, pulling him away from the ring toss, and made him get in line for the Hammer. Life is too short not to have fun, or for that matter, to drink bad wine.

* * *

Touch for Health is a remarkable self-help discipline. A practitioner tests the body's major muscle groups for initial strength. If a muscle group in an arm or leg is found to be weak, or unable to resist mild applied pressure, it is considered imbalanced. To remedy the situation, acupressure is used in specific areas, allowing energy to flow back into the muscle. Easy and effective, it is based on two main principles. One is acupuncture and meridian-balancing, as practiced in Oriental medicine. The other is Applied Kinesiology, the study of muscle groups and their movement and function. It is a powerful technique and I found it extremely beneficial in helping to improve my overall health and maintain a high level of visual function.

Meeting Dr. John Thie, the founder of Touch for Heath, was a great privilege. If he had been a medical doctor instead of a chiropractor, I'm sure his work would have gained the wide recognition it deserves. As it is, over one million people worldwide have taken a course in this remarkable self-help therapy. It quickly became an integral part of my own teaching.

Now I felt the program was complete. The years of experimentation and research were at an end. I had covered all bases. With this comprehensive approach, I was ready to go public. The time had come to give my work a clinical trial, a natural conclusion to the past ten years of experimentation.

No one else was offering either hope or a plan for improvement to those who suffered from serious eye disorders, and I could offer both. My personal success, going from being legally blind to being a legally licensed driver, was evidence enough for many people that the program worked. In addition, my son and those members of my family who were part of my research had all undergone positive change in their vision. I knew I should be able to duplicate the results with others. Because I learned one discipline at a time, the process of regaining most of my sight took years. I felt other people shouldn't require anywhere near so long to notice improvement.

Word spreads fast when something is working. My first call from overseas caught me on a day I was spending at home. It was from Spain; the man on the other end—a writer, an American who lived there—heard about me from a friend. His name was Jimmy. His sight was failing and he wanted to work on his eyes with me.

Here was someone willing to come nearly half way around the world to do my program. It was unnerving. My confidence flew out the window as I realized the enormous responsibility I had. Especially since I couldn't guarantee that anyone's vision would return, I had a hard time saying, "Sure, come on over."

I told Jimmy I truly didn't know if I could help him, but if he was willing to come to California—and not expect a fast fix—I would be more than happy to work with him. We exchanged addresses and phone numbers and he said he'd call back with information about when his plane would arrive in San Francisco. I said I'd pick him up.

He made it clear that he was a struggling author with a family to support. I understood and was happy to offer him a place to stay. That would ease the financial impact on him, and if he didn't do well, at least I wouldn't feel so guilty about the money he'd spent. Ru was happy to give up his bed and his room. It was the first of many times he did that so someone could attend my program.

Jimmy was the most lovable teddy bear of a man I'd ever met. At the airport, when Ru and I rescued him and his luggage, he looked utterly forlorn. Though he was exhausted from the long flight, we both felt like we were old friends, reuniting. On the way back to Novato, I decided to show him some of the sights of lower Marin. We went to Tiburon, a small European-style village situated on San Francisco Bay. Quaint little restaurants with decks going out over the water for their sun-loving clients lined the streets. We got a table overlooking the water with a magnificent view of the hills and cities that circle the Bay. Jimmy shared pictures of his family and told me of his vision problem in more detail.

His eyes were doing the exact opposite of what mine did. His central sight was impaired, making reading impossible. I was confused and thought maybe his diagnosis of retinitis pigmentosa had been a mistake. He assured me it was not, reminding me there were different types of RP. I knew he was right, but since mine started with the sides closing in, I tended to assume all types were the same, even if they had a few variations.

Because I'd not had the luxury of testing it on a large number of people, especially those with different types of RP, I was still very uncertain about what my program could do. Self-doubts surfaced, as I now faced my first client from out of the country.

In no way did I want to mislead or give false hope to someone experiencing serious eye problems. I knew only too well how demoralizing poor sight could be. In fact, depression seems to be common among people with limited sight. It's a physical and emotional depression that takes enormous effort to overcome and it never goes away completely. It lurks in the wings, barely out of reach, waiting only for a tiny signal to come rushing back into full view.

Jimmy was wonderful. He was willing to try all of my suggestions. We worked together during the day with the training and the therapies I had developed, then cooked dinner together. He loved to show us dishes he learned to cook in Spain. Afterwards we talked about anything and everything. He was trying with every ounce of determination to make a success of his trip and I found his willingness touching. His determination reminded me of my own struggle and that made us feel even closer.

One evening, a lecture on Holistic Health was scheduled at a health retreat called Forest Farms, in the hills of western Marin County, and Jimmy expressed an interest in going. I agreed to take him. By the time we were to leave, one of the worst storms in recent history was unleashing its fury. How we had the courage to undertake a trip over back roads I knew to be treacherous even in daylight is a mystery. That we reached our destination seemed a miracle.

I don't remember the meeting itself too well, but I do recall that by the time it was finished the rain had slowed to a gentle mist. Later, as we walked through the campgrounds to the parking area, we noticed a hot tub. A few people were enjoying the warmth and relaxation of the water. Jimmy, not having experienced a hot tub before, wanted to give it a try.

This was an outdoor, redwood barrel tub, with a crude step on the outside and no seats on the inside. Clothing was optional, although everyone was nude. Jimmy was an astonished but willing participant. We slipped behind the shower stall and undressed, shivering all the while. I hid behind Jimmy and we quickly got into the tub.

There seems to be a type of etiquette regarding the attitude of those who are already in the tub in relation to those who are getting in. You don't look at the person who, naked as a jaybird, is trying as gracefully as possible to climb into the barrel. Looking is only permitted once the person is tucked into the tub, with water up to his or her armpits. Jimmy and I tumbled into the water, splashing and creating a giant wave. Both of us had the same body type: round and fully packed. Of course, in my mind, I looked like Sophia Loren.

As it was Jimmy's first experience in a hot tub, I warned him that we mustn't stay too long. The heat can be dangerous if you're not accustomed to it. But he didn't care. He loved it and I'm sure, if he could, he would have stayed until sunup.

As we soaked, I thought back to an earlier time at this hilltop retreat when I had some enlightening experiences.

When I was trying to learn all I could about acupressure and shiatsu, I received a notice that a Japanese master teacher would be giving a weekend workshop at Forest Farms. Accommodations and meals were to be included, however the price was out of my range and budget. Any money I earned went quickly into raising a growing boy. No regrets—that was my priority and I never complained. However, with those self-imposed budgetary restrictions, I had to come up with creative ways to get what I wanted. That included extra courses on alternative medicine.

After a few days of creative thinking, I decided to call the retreat center to see if they needed any volunteer help with cleaning or kitchen work. They did and I was hired. I thought I could sneak a peek into the class on my breaks and perhaps pick up knowledge and techniques to help my eyesight. Besides, if I could get a minute alone with the instructor, I might ask about eyes and what to do for them. It wouldn't be too much to ask, I thought, justifying the boldness of my plan.

The first morning found me up to my elbows in the dirty pots and pans. I was the breakfast cleaner-upper. Over forty people were attending the conference and tons of dishes needed to be scrubbed clean. My hopes were being dashed as I plunged in to retrieve yet another dish. Maybe this hadn't been such a good idea after all. Oh well, I'd volunteered for the weekend and I wouldn't back out now.

After I washed what seemed to be a million dishes, the retreat supervisor asked me to take some sheets over to one of the cottages. I perked up considerably. The cottage that needed linen was right next to the conference hall where the course was in progress. Now would my luck hold? Could I sneak in and listen for a while, picking up pearls of wisdom?

Holding the sheets so as to give myself a look of belonging, I opened the door to the lecture hall.

I could see the instructor at the far end of the room talking to his students. I started to walk farther in and immediately tripped over something directly in my path. It was one of his students, sitting on a pillow, well out of my range of vision. As I stumbled, a chain reaction began, and by the time the fall was over, I managed to hit or roll over several students. Sheets went flying everywhere and the class came to a complete stop.

My face turned a deep shade of embarrassment colors. I was confused, stressed beyond imagination. My vision had diminished in response to the increased level of adrenaline, which was impairing blood circulation to my head. The teacher's voice was very deep and his demand brought me to full attention.

"Come here, young woman," he demanded. I wanted to speak to this master of Oriental techniques, but not like this. All I wanted now was to disappear.

People helped pick up the linen I'd tossed around like the makings of a giant Caesar salad. By the time I worked my way to the front, the entire room was silent. The class must be thinking I was in big trouble. I certainly did. That's what I got for trying to be slick. Trying to get something free. Well, not exactly free. After all, I was willing to work.

The closer I got, the clearer I saw his face. It was kind and gentle. I began to relax. He reached out and took my hand, pulling me to his side. He asked me my name and I mumbled a reply. He held my wrist while we talked and, within a few minutes, told the class I had a serious eye problem and couldn't see very well. He asked me if I was one of his students who had come in late. Oh, to be so embarrassed and in shock at the same time!

But how did he know I had eye problems? He wasn't a sorcerer (as I first imagined). His ability to recognize my problem was based on his observation of my theatrical entrance and his study of "wrist pulse" diagnosis. I blurted out the story of how I couldn't attend due to financial considerations and how I volunteered to work, hopefully to glean a few morsels of knowledge. He relaxed his hold on my wrist and told me to sit down. Asking that several students move aside, he said he wanted me to remain right in front, which gave me the best seat in the house.

From then on, I was not only a student, but the official guinea pig. Whenever our illustrious instructor needed to demonstrate the application of acupressure, he used me. I was in hog heaven. Not only was I learning, but the master himself was actually working on me. Me! Truly it was a gift from the Universe.

❦

My memory of that time faded as my attention returned to the hot tub and Jimmy. It had been a magical experience then, and now here I was again, still benefiting from what this place offered. The two of us, Jimmy and I, were sitting in the hot tub, enjoying the remainder of the evening. Jimmy felt he could see a little better when he was in the hot water. That had a certain logic to me, since vision is affected by stress and the hot tub certainly does reduce stress. This type of therapy had been used in the Orient for centuries. Had I stumbled onto a new component for my program? I decided to find other such places that were a little more accessible, for Jimmy and me to try out.

There was a health center in Cotati, a small town up the highway from Novato. Cotati was a radical place, way ahead of its time. I found out that Jimmy and I could use their facility for the nominal fee of a dollar per person, per hour. It fit our budget so off we went, this time during the day.

It had two tubs. One was indoors, a built-in tile Jacuzzi, with lots of jets swirling the hot water in miniature whirlpools. The other was a redwood barrel, similar to the one we were in at Forest Farms. Jimmy and I chose the indoor tub, as it looked like it had more jets. We liked the feel of the jets, massaging the muscles and melting away tension. Clothing was optional, but Jimmy and I came prepared. We were the only two in the tub with suits on. That was fine with us. Naked at night is okay, especially if you don't see well in the dark. Here, in broad daylight, our being dressed seemed more appropriate. Besides, this was a professional experiment with the aim of improving our sight. And, if it didn't help, at least we got clean and relaxed at the same time. So we were both enjoying the water therapy, when suddenly I heard him gasp, "Oh, my God!"

He nodded wordlessly in the direction of the stairs leading into the Jacuzzi. I looked and saw a beautiful, tall, blonde woman, stark naked, descending into the water. Jimmy, over the noise of the gurgling bubbles, was whispering to me that she was the most beautiful woman he had ever seen. I had to agree that she was also the most attractive naked woman I had ever seen. Not that I have seen that many, but she was exceptionally lovely.

Then it dawned on me—Jimmy had seen her, seen her centrally and well enough to notice her stunning beauty. We were euphoric and started giggling like a couple of kids. In this giddy mood, we started fantasizing about an addition to my course—a hot tub for men with a gorgeous woman and one with an equally sexy hunk for the women. We knew the American Medical Association would never endorse such shenanigans, but we had a lot of laughs kicking the idea around.

I wondered how Jimmy would tell his wife about what stimulated the improvement of his vision. "Well, dear, you see, I was receiving hydrotherapy when a visual stimulant of perfection and enormous beauty opened my central sight." Okay, I'd go for that explanation. But would a wife?

Unfortunately, Jimmy's improvement wasn't great, even though it was tremendously exciting for us both to experience. We became close and I loved him as a brother, so I was crushed when his sight didn't improve greatly. I hoped, of course, that he would regain all his vision, but that was not to be. I know he was disappointed, but I don't know if he knew how disappointed I was. I almost quit after Jimmy. I didn't want to face another human being who tried so hard and didn't get the desired results.

Jimmy was the first person with a complex vision problem who traveled such a long distance to see me. My confidence was shot. It was a difficult lesson for me to swallow. But at least he had some personal success, since, while he was working with me in California, his agent made a good deal on his book.

⚬⚬⚬

Not long afterward, the same week Northern California got shaken up by a 4.9 quake, I got a new RP client. Her name was Susan, a student at Sacramento State University. She was a beautiful young woman, about twenty years old. Her doctors recently told her she had retinitis pigmentosa and would go blind. Her life was demolished by that news, and she had no idea what to do. She was an extremely talented pianist, her education was nearly complete, and her goal was to teach music. She was engaged, but after hearing her doctor's predictions, she was confused about having children. She might even call off her marriage. It was a terrible crisis for her.

Susan liked the idea of working on her eyes. It gave her hope and options, options the traditional doctors didn't offer. She and her father drove down from Sacramento twice a week to work with me. I started her on the regimen a little at a time, and within four months she noticed a distinct change in her ability to play the piano and get around the college campus. She and her fiancé even went dancing. Her sight, tested by an independent doctor, showed marked improvement. Not only was I thrilled for her, but also my self-confidence returned.

With that success under my belt, I felt sure the time had come to go public. Speaking engagements were one way I could get the message out. My past work experience with Connections taught me how to get the public's attention. It was an easy task, starting with lining up speeches at local community organizations, including the senior citizens' centers in several cities.

I felt the time had also come to look into getting information published in local newspapers and, perhaps, in a magazine. Never having written an article or even a query letter, I looked in the Yellow Pages for help.

Marin County prides itself as an area where many hundreds of published authors reside, a large percentage of whom live in the town of Mill Valley. So finding a writer in the area was easy. The difficult part was choosing which one. I finally decided to work with a young writer named Alice. She was very helpful and our article was accepted by a national magazine, Let's Live. It had a significant circulation among people interested in natural health. It was a perfect outlet for my story.

The magazine was going to release the article, with the title "Learning to See Again," in its 50th Anniversary issue, in January 1983. Knowing I would have national exposure, I recognized the need to make plans for handling the potential response. And…the time had come to move again.

❦

The thought of having people arrive from all over the country to participate in my program presented new and interesting challenges. Novato, a sleepy little bedroom community thirty minutes north of San Francisco, had only one hotel and poor public transportation. I doubted it would be satisfactory for my needs. Also, to make the program available, I knew I must keep my overhead down, so people could afford it.

I already discovered that transportation costs alone sometimes exceeded the fee I charged for the program. My being sensitive to economic realities was necessary, as many people I worked with were on fixed incomes because of age or as a result of being legally blind, which often meant they were unable to secure decent-paying jobs. I needed to find a place close to inexpensive rental housing and, also, either within walking distance of or with easy access to public transportation.

My Irish luck seemed to be holding firm. I had developed a program that could help people's sight improve, but my clients were usually poor. Nevertheless, the real rewards came from seeing them get better. Money can only be spent, but knowing these people were reading four or five lines farther down the chart than they could just a few weeks earlier had more value to me than money. Anyway, I realized early on that I wasn't going to get rich from doing this. Often, when circumstances warranted, I even gave the program for nothing, since my need to help people improve their sight came ahead of my need for money. I had to charge fees to be able to live and raise my son, but doing so was never my priority.

❦

The solution to my dilemma was moving to Guerneville, a resort community on the Russian River west of Santa Rosa. It was thirty miles north of Novato in a beautiful part of the country. Its hills, redwood trees, and a lazy river winding down to the Pacific Ocean made the decision easy.

Being in Guerneville was going to be like living in a vacationland all year. Since it had a tourist-based economy, housing prices were reasonable, especially in the off-season. There were many rentals and hotels around the area, providing economical options for potential clients traveling from afar. Ru and I moved to Guerneville shortly after Christmas 1982.

A big blue two-story Victorian house complete with an old-fashioned front porch was waiting for us. It provided sufficient room for us to live in and was big enough so I could do my work without leaving home.

After getting the boxes and furniture moved in, we paused as the day came to an end. Friends who had helped us move were gone; Ru and I were alone in our new house. It was time to turn on the lights. The sky was overcast and rain had fallen off and on all day, filling the town's overflowing creeks and the river even more.

The lights didn't work. The flood had taken its toll on Pacific Gas and Electric, and here we were in a new house, with boxes all over the place and no electricity.

Oh well, Ru and I had camped out before. By the time darkness came, we were prepared for the night. Sleeping bags on my double-bed mattress near the fireplace would keep us cozy and warm. Fortunately, plenty of wood was available for the large stone fireplace, which was used originally for heating the whole house. It was very effective this particular evening.

We had hot dogs and all the other picnic fixings necessary for preparing tube steaks. Straightened coat hangers made nifty hot dog warmers for the fire. Ru found the checkerboard. We played, ate, and shared scary ghost stories until, exhausted, we fell into a sound sleep. It was a wonderful way to spend the first night in our new home.

We were back in a country setting, complete with a magnificent view of mountains and forests. Less than a mile down the road was Armstrong Woods, a state park with virgin redwoods. Some of its trees were over two thousand years old. Hugging a tree again felt good. Yet, in our new location, we were only a short walk along a paved road from a pizza parlor, the main street of town and, for Ru, a video game arcade. He was in heaven. This little resort community was a tenth the size of Novato, yet had more things available for us to do and we didn't need the car.

My article in Let's Live finally came out. Within several weeks, nearly a hundred letters had arrived asking for more information. It was very exciting and most of my time was spent reading and answering these sometimes heartbreaking requests. Before long, I scheduled my first class, having decided to try a small group of people, teaching them all at once. Until now, I always worked on a one-to-one basis, repeating to a current client exactly what I said to another client an hour before. I finally realized that a group would be a much more efficient way to share my program.

While waiting for the magazine article to come out, I developed a workbook. I recognized that in order to teach in a class setting, I needed to organize the material and to offer participants something to take home when they left. Mine was a long-term, self-help therapy program, so having a good reference book made sense. I hired a professional photographer to take pictures of the exercises and acupressure points I discussed in the program and was ready to go. But when the printer told me how much reproducing photographs would cost, I nearly fainted dead away. Using photos, I realized clearly, was out of the question. Now what was I to do?

I decided to learn to draw and illustrate the book myself! It made logical sense. Thus, without knowing what was involved, I stocked up on drawing-instruction books, as well as the required pens, pencils, and papers. Nothing was too difficult for me. Learning not to set limitations for Ru taught me the same for myself. If I believed I could do it, then it would get done.

Wrong.

It was very, very difficult, and I was not at all pleased with my early attempts to draw. This was going to take much longer than I thought, and I'd need to spend most of my time working on the illustrations. Keeping the house organized and preparing meals, I realized, was taking far too many of the hours I could be using to finish the book.

We had an extra bedroom, so I decided to advertise for someone to help me. I placed an ad in the next day's paper. In exchange for room and board, someone could help clean the house and cook for the two of us. That way, I could do the book in no time.

The first person to call was a woman who sounded young and enthusiastic. She was looking for a place to live while she worked part-time. Her passion was learning to make Celtic harps and, as luck would have it, the only factory making these harps was less than a mile from our house. I liked the way she sounded; she seemed very personable. Thus, the job was filled and she moved in that afternoon.

I'd learned a while back to be careful what I wish for. If I was clear about what I wanted, I usually got it quickly. This seemed to be one of those times. However, the Universe also had a few tricks up its sleeve.

The three of us enjoyed a tasty dinner, one we all prepared together, to celebrate Maxine's arrival. I could tell that Ru liked Maxine and she took to him immediately. I knew this was going to go well. That mealtime also provided a chance for Maxine and me to get to know each other better. We sat down with a cup of tea to talk while Ru, with school the next day, prepared for bed.

She finally got around to asking me why I needed a mother's helper. I'd already told her I had a project to complete. Since I was feeling more comfortable with her, I disclosed my plans in more detail.

She listened intently as I discussed my eye problem and the program I had developed to improve sight. She was amazed and said she couldn't tell I had a vision problem at all. I was pleased with her comment. Indeed my sight was much better, though I still had a few difficulties, especially at night.

Then I told her of my decision to learn to draw and illustrate the workbook myself. Her mouth dropped open. It turned out she was a graduate of the Art Department at UCLA, with specialties in drawing and illustration. Once again the Universe heard my request for help. Here, thank you, was Maxine.

So I cooked the meals, cleaned the house, and did all the menial labor. Maxine, in exchange for room and board, did the drawings. She was fabulous and very quick. My workbook was at the printer within the month. Life was very good to us. We were additionally blessed to hear Celtic harp music, played by my resident artist. What more could one want?

Three students were in my first class—two ladies, both in their sixties, and a gentleman from Oregon who claimed to be eighty-two. It went as smooth as glass—except for the time I lost my patience with one of the ladies who had an annoying habit of interrupting anyone who was talking. Her questions were often inane and not related to the conversation.

Finally, her interruptions sent me running from the room and, in a childish outburst, I slammed the door as hard as I could. As soon as the echo of the slam died down, I realized my gross error. I was the teacher and this was my house. Sitting in the living room were three people who paid me to teach them the technique I developed to improve sight. There was no way out of it. I had to calm down, collect myself, and go back in there. They were waiting for me to finish.

No one said a word and the woman whose behavior led to my acting like an idiot didn't interrupt for the rest of the day. I had a lot to learn, and these early sessions, while often embarrassing, were very educational. The other two people took me aside later and said they understood. If I hadn't jumped up so suddenly and left the room, they said they would have done so themselves. That made me feel a little better.

The town we had moved to was quaint, with strange undercurrents. After arriving there, I found out numerous changes had taken place on the Russian River since my visits as a teenager. Many of the resorts had been bought by gay men and women from San Francisco, turning the resort town into a retreat for gays on the weekends. The townspeople were clearly divided. The money the gays brought into the community was helpful, but it was supporting the gay resorts, not the family-oriented resorts. The specter of AIDS had started to make its way into the public eye. The ignorance of AIDS and, in general, of the gay community by straights caused a great deal of stress. My clients, coming from such places as Kansas, Montana, and Iowa, didn't understand what was happening. They did express their concerns about the possibility of contracting AIDS from the drinking water, as well as from the swimming pools. We still didn't know much about the disease in the early Eighties.

As much as I loved living in the woods and river area, I decided to move to Santa Rosa, a larger, family-oriented city, where my clients would feel more comfortable. Santa Rosa is a beautiful city, surrounded by hills. It's rustic, but classy. The prices were a little higher, but people had much more to see and do.

Since I had about a year's worth of clients lined up, I felt secure in putting money into leasing a house. The house I found had a circular drive, a wall-sized brick fireplace, landscaped front and back yards, and a swimming pool with diving board. It was completely furnished in an elegant style. The bonus was a cottage on the grounds, perfect for my work with clients. It was expensive, but why not? I felt like a million dollars, doing my work and living in a swank place.

Playing the rich lady was a lot of fun. Ru adjusted just fine and loved to swim every day. We began to have parties—outdoors when the weather was beautiful and indoors when it wasn't. This was the first house I could entertain in. And I found out how many of my friends like to swim. They seemed to come out of the woodwork, especially when the temperature climbed to the ninety-degree mark. We were having the time of our lives, Ru and I.

Time was proving my program a success. I still had doubts, but I was gaining confidence with each person who completed the course and reported good news. Now the point had come for us to get serious about gathering the data for research. The words of that pompous research scientist surfaced frequently in my mind. He had stated unequivocally that unless I could provide clinical proof that the program worked, it would never become part of any serious treatment modality for eye problems.

The obvious answer was to start a nonprofit organization. I could raise funds from the general public as well as from major corporations, and everything would be tax-deductible to the donors. I felt that would solve all the problems I saw coming up. I could still offer the program, particularly to people who couldn't afford it, without taking a bath financially. And I could get funding to help support the research I needed to document the program properly. It made sense. But how was I going to start a nonprofit business? As I had in the past, I got a book to teach me what I needed to learn. Since I had been successful at most things I tried in the past ten years, I felt I could learn a new game. After all, how hard could it be?

12

LIGHTS, CAMERA, ACTION

Somewhere along the road, the idea that I could do anything if I put my mind to it got embedded in my brain. At that moment, the concept of starting a nonprofit corporation appeared to be the most logical approach to solving my problem. Under a nonprofit umbrella, we could raise funds to help supplement our services. People otherwise unable to attend could be helped. Funding from individuals and from government sources would provide the money we needed to fully document the results.

Finding what I needed at the bookstore was easy. Right next to the Do-It-Yourself Wills and Do-It-Yourself For-Profit Corporation books were the Do-It-Yourself Nonprofit Corporation books. I found the forms I needed for submission to various local, State, and Federal agencies. For twenty dollars and change, anyone could build a dream. Anyone who understands the instructions, that is. They're the hard part.

The difficulty wasn't only in interpreting the lingo of the book. After hours of straining, I was having trouble seeing the words on the page. Sunlight had become oppressive and painful, causing me to wear sunglasses more than usual. I had been noticing tiny black dots floating in my central vision, and a warning bell sounded deep in my mind, but I buried it quickly. Instead, I made excuses. Time to get an eye exam. It had been a while. Back to my friendly optometrist, Larry Jebrock. Time to get a new pair of reading glasses, that's all. Anyway, I trusted Larry's judgment. No one I had gone to in the past could create a prescription for clear sight any better than Larry.

Visiting my old friends was exciting. Their office sounded busy, a good sign things were going well. Larry was interested to hear what I had been doing. He nodded in agreement, liking my plans for a nonprofit organization. "Perfect solution," he said, as he started to examine my eyes.

Immediately I knew something was wrong. Larry was a straightforward doctor. With the most compassion I had ever heard in his voice, he told me he detected subtle evidence that cataracts were developing. I couldn't believe it. A serious setback for my eyesight, just as my vision had been doing so well.

Almost ninety percent of people diagnosed with RP had early cataracts. I knew that. Thinking I had been one of the ten percent not to have cataracts, I was surprised by Larry's observation. The cataracts associated with retinitis pigmentosa, which come on dead-center and affect central reading ability immediately by blocking light, are different from those that form in the elderly (which do not usually interfere with central sight until their advanced stages). The centrally located cataract not only obstructs light entering the eye but also causes it to bounce around and strike areas which are not designed for such intensity. That was what had been causing my increasing sensitivity to sunlight. Knowing this didn't make things easier. It was, in fact, a shock to my head and heart.

It felt as though I had been hit by the same truck for the second time. Now what would happen? My emotions were all over the place, bouncing off the walls, slamming into the ceiling. Why had I bothered to try so hard to improve my sight? All along, these time bombs were living in my lenses, waiting to blow up.

Well, if anyone had to tell me the bad news, I'm glad it was Larry. His concern was genuine, but more than that, he got back in balance a lot faster than I did. "What are you going to do about your eyes now?"

At first I thought his question insensitive and inappropriate. I almost hated him for a second. Didn't he realize cataracts would cause me to go completely blind?

Of course he did. But he was a fighter too, and he provided a hard push to bring back the rebel inside me. All it meant was that I would have to work harder with this new challenge. I became lazy after the progress I made in the past. Now I had a pressing need for more research and experimentation. Back to the drawing board.

Nevertheless, my mood was a shade deeper than midnight black. I felt as though a crushing weight had been placed on my shoulders, and I seriously doubted whether I could carry the burden. A deep well of self-pity overflowed into my entire being. Hugging Ru for dear life was the only thing that kept me from going off the deep end. He was there for me, unquestioning and totally giving.

He was scared. It wasn't like Mom to be so frightened, so depressed, crying like this. I knew it wasn't fair to him, but I didn't have anyone else to turn to; besides, he knew more about my struggle for sight than anyone else in the world. Ru had been through it all and now he was comforting me, telling me, "It'll be okay, Mom. Just do your program." My twelve-year-old son was my parent at that moment. His love was my only lifeline to reality.

❦

Bouncing back from blows like this new one was getting harder and harder, but after a few weeks I began to look at the bright side. Hey, maybe I could find something that would help myself and others deal with cataracts. Something out there had to work. All I needed was to discover more about cataracts, then look into finding a cure or a therapy. As long as I had a plan, my emotions could stabilize themselves.

Meanwhile, back at the nonprofit ranch, our paperwork was being completed and filed. I had a great deal of help from, guess who? Kathleen. Since my ability to read was compromised, my dear sister came to the rescue. Her help got the paperwork finished within a relatively short period of time. It was easier than I had imagined. Of course, that's because Kathleen did the hard part.

The Let's Live article was still bringing in some clients, three and four at a time. I was perfecting the group teaching and therapy approach. The financial input of these clients made it possible for us to stay at the luxurious home we were leasing. We became spoiled by having friends and family over for the weekend barbecues.

One weekend my mother dropped in unexpectedly. She and I were getting closer after having been estranged for many years. During those horrible times when I was a teenager, I treated her pretty badly. Now that I was a mom, I felt guilty for what I had done. I did not want to hurt her anymore, though I'm sure she feared I would if she got too close.

But during the past few years, as I'd searched for therapies that would help RP, Mom became my number-one guinea pig and supporter. Her feedback was of tremendous value. I wouldn't have done as well without her help.

This particular evening was warm, with the scent of honeysuckle floating in the air. Our guests had gone and the pool finally calmed down, reflecting the night lights brilliantly. Mom and I were sitting by the pool, sipping some wine. We were both happy as the cement beneath us radiated a warmth absorbed from the hot sun, adding to our total relaxation.

She and I began to talk about the pain and frustration of what happened when I was a runaway teenager. Now that I had a child nearing his teens, I couldn't imagine how I would live if Ru ran away. How she had managed to survive, I just didn't know. Of course, she had other kids to worry about and couldn't fall apart because of my stupidity. Regardless, it was the first time we'd talked about the past like this. I felt years of guilt and hard feelings peeling away.

I had never asked Mom about her childhood. When she started telling me of her youth, about growing up in the hills of Kentucky and West Virginia, about her hopes and dreams, I got an entirely different picture of her. She told me she wanted to be a writer...of science fiction. I was astonished. For as long as I could remember—well, at least for the past fifteen years—I wanted to be a writer. My favorite books from the age of twelve to eighteen were science fiction. I couldn't believe the connections we had! Mom even started writing a book about outer space and UFOs when she was a teenager. Go figure. My mom? This was great. We had broken new ground. Sharing secret fantasies and dreams, we were becoming good friends. It was the start of a new phase of our relationship.

Mom was glad I was forming the nonprofit program and offered her support. My heart swelled with love and pride that wonderful warm summer evening when I rediscovered my mother and gained a friend.

❦

My looking for answers about cataracts was a time-consuming project. Some might even have thought it a hopeless one, since the official medical establishment, with all of its power and funding, was doing the same thing. But I was coming at the matter from a different perspective. I had the cataracts and that gave me an edge over any scientist researching the matter objectively. Also, I knew the situation from an inner point of view and that tended to stimulate my intuition in the direction of a solution. With my knowledge of alternative therapies, I could easily think in terms of different approaches. So it was at least worth a try. I had nothing to lose and a lot to gain. Besides, my personal experience with confronting eye disease included a certain degree of success.

To review the literature about cataracts, I got a large magnifying glass and started reading. One of the first things I found out was that there are many different types, so finding an easy answer didn't appear likely. I discovered the kind I had was specific to retinitis pigmentosa; however, there was little more information on them. What I did find was not encouraging. Research indicated that many people develop cataracts as a complication of RP. Apparently, medical doctors had not given much attention to this complication. Their attitude seemed to me to be, "Why bother operating on the cataracts, when the patient will go blind anyway?"

My blood began to boil as I realized that countless thousands of people might have gone blind needlessly because of an ignorant prejudice on their doctor's part. RP itself usually affects side vision and night vision—not central vision, or at least not until the final stages. For some, that stage may take twenty or thirty years to develop. However, a central cataract, specific to RP, affects central sight almost immediately. So people were allowed to go blind from the cataract—a problem that could have been solved—and lose many years of potential sightedness. I had already seen limited belief systems, prejudices, and closed-minded attitudes put people into little boxes, and now I was seeing it again.

The genetic eye disease retinitis pigmentosa did not have a cure. (The work I had done with

RP produced no "cures," nor did I ever claim that. People improved their vision, but no one—including me—actually cured or got rid of the eye disease. To me, a cure means you don't have the problem anymore.) Cataracts, however, did have a cure. Surgery, I discovered, could help. That was encouraging. If I couldn't find something less radical, at least hope was available in the form of surgery and lens implants.

Most of the alternative methods I applied didn't help the cataracts. Many, like putting honey in my eyes at bedtime, didn't make any sense at all, although I was willing to try them. The honey, for example, stung like crazy and blurred my vision for nearly three days. I didn't try it more than once. My instinct was that it wasn't a good thing to do to the eyes. Remember, I had my standards. If it feels good, do it. If it doesn't, then don't do it again. That was my motto and I lived by it.

Some parts of my program did make life easier. Color therapy, I discovered, helped relieve the stress and light sensitivity, so I began doing it morning and night—for about twenty minutes at a time.

In the end, I got the lens implant surgery. I found the best surgeon in Northern California. He felt I would be helped by the surgery and was willing to do it. He didn't agree with the doctors who wouldn't touch a patient with RP, the ones who thought, "Why bother, they're going blind anyway."

That attitude made him as angry as it made me. I liked this doctor. Most of all, I trusted him.

He was fantastic! If I had known what the process was like, I wouldn't have been so frightened, so depressed, so desperate to find an alternative. He was a consummate surgeon. "Only the best" was his motto. He had built an outpatient surgical center in his office, where he could control the environment and other conditions with great precision. That was better than working out of an operating room in the local hospital. There is always a risk of something going wrong, so don't misunderstand me. I was plenty worried. After all, these eyes are not replaceable. One slip and they could be gone. However, getting a great surgeon increased the odds dramatically in my favor.

The surgery was over in forty minutes. I had been awake, but heavily drugged with an intravenous dose of Valium. The nerve-block injection (the most painful part of the procedure) temporarily paralyzed my eyeball. Only one eye is operated on at a time. It's better that way, in case something goes wrong. My right eye had been operated on first, since it was my weakest. A large bandage covered the eye protector I would wear until my doctor-visit the next morning.

The nurse gave me a small brown envelope as I was leaving the surgery recovery room. Inside, she told me, were several pain pills and one sleeping pill. As I began to protest that I didn't take sleeping pills, she told me to take it later to make sure I got a good night's sleep. She pointed out the doctor's home phone number on the back of the envelope. "If something is wrong, he wants to know right away. Don't hesitate calling him, any time of the night, if you really need to," were her parting instructions. I never heard of such a thing. Normally I would have to call the doctor's answering service, which would track him down for me, asking him to call back. Not my doctor. He went home from the office on surgery days and didn't leave until time to report back to the office. He was a dedicated physician—a nonsmoker and a nondrinker, who even avoided caffeine to prevent hand tremors.

I was home by noon, the pain hit as the muscles around my eyes came back to life. That's what hurt the most, the muscles in the lid and eyebrow area. The eyeball itself doesn't have much feeling. The cornea, the clear part that covers the iris, or colored part, is the only area with sensitive tissue. So my eye itself didn't hurt, but the surrounding areas were in a total muscle spasm.

My sister Kellee brought me in for my checkup. No one really is sure whether eye surgery is a success until the bandage comes off. The unveiling of my eye was to be the highlight of the whole process. Oh, the doctor can say it went well, but the proof is in the seeing. Needless to say, I was a nervous wreck.

Kellee was looking good that day, as she always did. I was continuingly amazed at how she learned to accessorize her outfits with inexpensive but great-looking earrings, bracelets and, when appropriate, necklaces. I had a lot to learn from this one.

She could tell I was nervous, and as I sat in the exam chair waiting for the doctor to come in, she decided to tell me a joke.

"Did you hear the one about the blind guy who went into a bar?"

I couldn't believe my ears. Here we were, waiting to see if I was blind or not, and this dipsy doodle was going to tell me a blind-guy joke. Oh well, I figured I might as well go along with her, because I knew from past experience that you can't put my little sister off for long. She gets her way, sooner or later.

"No, I didn't," I said, giving her the go-ahead sign. Without it, you can't really tell a joke. It's like a "knock-knock" joke. If someone doesn't say, "Who's there?" there's no joke.

Kellee grinned and started in. "This guy walks into a bar with his guide dog. A big German Shepherd. The blind guy bends down and picks up his dog by the tail and starts swinging him around his head. He swings the dog around about five times. The bartender sees this and jumps over the bar, yelling at the blind guy. 'Hey buddy, what the hell are you doing to that poor dog?' The blind guy puts his dog down, turns to the bartender, and says, 'I was just looking around.' "

Well, it was funny. Even with one eye bandaged, not knowing if I was blind or not, I laughed hysterically. Thank God Kellee had brought me for the checkup. Her sense of timing and humor took my mind off my precarious condition. By the time the doctor walked into the room, Kellee and I were hurting from laughing so hard.

The doctor was chuckling as he began taking my bandage off. "Well," he said, "I've seen and heard it all now. This is the first time I have had a patient laugh while waiting to get the bandage off."

The bandage was removed. My eye felt swollen and funny. As that eye, my right eye, adjusted to the light in the room, I raised my hand in front of it. Tears of happiness and gratitude began welling up—in both eyes. I could see the lines on my hand, the ridges that surround the joints of the fingers. I hadn't seen details like that in a long, long time.

I looked at Kellee, who was sitting anxiously on the couch across from the exam chair. I could see the color of her eyes, even the laugh lines. It was amazing. I had been looking at life as if it were a Doris Day movie, pretty but out of focus, as though Vaseline were smeared on the lens. Of course, the good thing was that I hadn't seen any blemishes or evidences of aging on the faces of my friends. Now I relished each line and blotchy skin area, everything tiny that had been beyond my visual capability. The surgery had been a success. Within a few months, I would get the left eye done, and then—watch my smoke. My sight was going to be perfect!

AMAZING GRACE

13

OPEN FOR BUSINESS

The approval for our nonprofit corporation came through with no problem. That meant we could seek funding to support the work. And getting public exposure with the local media was now much easier. Before I knew it, we were asked to be on one of the most popular live television shows in the Bay Area, "People Are Talking."

The show, hosted by Ann Franzer and Ross McGowan, aired live from San Francisco at ten in the morning, five days a week. It was an hour long and had some 200 people in the live studio audience. I was to be on first, with another guest scheduled for the second half. Optometrists Dr. Gregory King and Dr. Elliot Kaplan came with me to verify the results we had been achieving.

If anyone had taken my blood pressure or pulse rate as the show got underway, I think they'd have made a 911 call right there on live TV. To say I was nervous is to say that the sun is hot. A few minutes after I went on, however, I'd forgotten my rapid heartbeat and was totally involved in the show. I loved being on live television and felt I did a good job of explaining the program. The audience was laughing and applauding me at the most wonderful places. It went so well that the producer gave the entire hour to my interview, asking the other guest to come back at another time. It was exhilarating and went all too fast. (One woman in the studio audience inspired me by asking if I had written a book. I said no, but told her I was going to go home that very day and write one. Well, this is it.)

After the show, we received hundreds of calls asking for more information about my program and the work we were doing. It was my big debut and it went very well. A piece of cake, and I felt like the "actress" in me had been unleashed. Our organization was up and running, with a list of potential clients wanting to attend courses during the next six months. That one show paved the way for a lot of work for us. We were very satisfied.

❦

The name of our new organization was the hardest thing to decide on. Finally, I came up with Center for Eye Health Education. By this time, a suite of offices had materialized and the beginnings of a small staff were falling in place.

My idea was teaching the program in components, providing extensive therapy and education during a two- to three-week course. Clients would pay on a sliding scale basis, attending therapy sessions five days a week. Group sessions would enable clients to learn the home self-help program. Group time also afforded us the opportunity to talk about the personal and emotional problems associated with loss of sight.

It was a tremendously powerful vision program. My staff, who were all experts in their own field, were now eager to learn the programs I was teaching. They really took on the job of helping people. My vision was back, better than ever, and my center was a reality. The Universe was kind to me. When it knocked me down, it usually picked me up and put me in a better place. Prayers of thanks and gratitude were on my lips daily. Ru was healthy and the sun shone most days. Who could ask for more?

Within the year, we had two acupuncturists, a full-time acupressure massage technician, and a biofeedback therapist working with clients. My own time with the people had been cut to a few hours a day for group therapy. Administrative duties, fund raising, grant proposal writing, and public outreach demanded my attention. However, I made sure the care the participants were receiving achieved the desired results. We hired two optometrists to consult with the program and to record examinations before participants began, and to do follow-up exams on the last day of their stay.

The optometrists—Drs. King and Kaplan— scheduled examinations according to our course attendance. Both were wonderfully helpful and established excellent "before and after" testing, standardizing the tests so they would show any changes that took place. I watched those tests on the last day like a chicken hawk keeps an eye on dinner. They were my guidelines for judging if the program was successful.

The staff was doing a terrific job and I was extremely happy with the situation. Unfortunately I wasn't totally comfortable with administrative duties. My background wasn't in business, which was a drawback with regard to my being Executive Director. I did my best, but that wasn't good enough in the final analysis.

The "People Are Talking" show aired in August 1984. It, in turn, caught the attention of a television producer with access to a larger market. "Evening Magazine," a nationally syndicated television show, contacted the Center wanting to do a piece for their program. The segment on my work was to be only four and a half minutes long, but would air in eighty-five cities nationwide!

With all that attention, my getting a swollen head was not impossible, but my sisters Kathleen and Kellee were working with me, doing their best to keep my feet on the ground. Ru was taking all the publicity in stride. He confided in me that he knew all along I would become famous. Of course, he probably got that idea as a result of things I told him when he was just a young kid.

I also knew I was leaving a giant trail for my daughter to follow when she turned eighteen. That was never far from my thoughts and I was always aware that the more exposure I got, the easier her search would be.

The publicity wasn't just for me. It was for all those people who were told nothing could be done, who accepted blindness, gave up, and got lost in the medical shuffle. They had a chance to hear the truth: your situation is not hopeless.

Each time I saw clinical improvements, my determination became stronger for our program to be successful. Not because it was my program. It was their program. They made it work. They were the pioneers. They were the most courageous people I ever met. They often came to the program against their doctors' advice, even against the advice of their own families. I admired their strength.

I also found that my clients had a bond deeper than just one of impaired vision. All of them believed, deep down, that something, somewhere could help them. They were the ones who, after the initial shock of being told they were going blind, bounced back. My work was made easy by their openness and willingness to do what was necessary. I tried never to give false hope or mislead anyone. But the fact was: I was much better, and so were members of my own family. And now, with the help of the people who came to the Center, we were amassing case histories to demonstrate that these were not isolated, "freak" improvements, but ones that could be repeated over and over.

Not everyone improved, however, and I suffered deeply when brave people, expecting to be healed, weren't. We needed to know why they weren't, and the need for a thorough evaluation of our techniques and therapies haunted my waking hours. I began to write to foundations who studied and researched retinitis pigmentosa, requesting that they conduct independent evaluations of our work. Such evaluations could provide us with important answers. We might find out why some people regained a great deal of sight, while others experienced no change at all. Maybe the ones who didn't respond so dramatically needed more of a particular therapy or less of another. Without knowledge gained through those kinds of evaluations, I would never be able to refine our program so we could help all the people who needed it.

But the foundations did not respond to my pleas. Their reasons were not mysterious to me. Well-funded, highly publicized foundations must take a rigorously scientific approach to their research if they expect to stay in business. They cannot, in general, abandon mainstream methods and expect their mainstream funding to continue. It's a situation that tends to exclude more informal, homegrown approaches, the kind I had been taking. I did not really expect them to respond favorably to our work, but I didn't want to ignore the possibility that they might.

In the meantime, we continuingly acknowledged that this program was not a cure, though we definitely were getting improvements. Fortunately, those people who improved were in the majority, but that didn't make the failures any easier. I wanted desperately to have everyone get positive results.

◎❧

The newspaper, magazine, and television exposure brought letters and calls from all over the country. Inquiries from other countries began to come in the mail. We hadn't received any grants or public funding yet, but the influx of clients enabled us to keep the doors open and pay the staff salaries regularly. That was a success in itself.

My duties now included trying to find a way to independently determine the results of the program. The studies we accumulated were ignored by the medical profession. Their internal prejudices came pouring out when they discovered optometrists, not ophthalmologists, had done the before-and-after evaluations. They dismissed the studies as inconclusive and subjective. What they wanted was "objectivity," which I had done my best to provide. What they also wanted was to have data that had been collected by ophthalmologists. Actually, they didn't want me to demonstrate anything. I was mainly an irritation to them.

Now that did present a problem. First of all, without even thinking about what a thorough ophthalmological examination would cost (three to four times what an optometrist charges), just getting an ophthalmologist to be involved would be harder than winning the lottery. Managing the logistics of having one available to meet our schedule would be next to impossible. Since our clients came from all over and only stayed two or three weeks, the doctor would just about have to clear his own busy schedule and become available to us full-time. Normally an appointment for an ophthalmologist must be scheduled up to three months in advance. My chances of finding someone inclined to adapt to our circumstances were slim to none.

I was willing to comply with the requirement that our program be tested by the appropriate medically trained people, but I just didn't have the resources to gather the required documentation. We had to receive funding before we could do the impossible. The Catch-22 of all this was that getting the funding without a medical study would be next to impossible. The maze of confusion between funding and AMA practices was making me crazy. The only thing that kept me at it was the people. We were meeting and working with the most wonderful people in the world.

⟨⟩

While all of that was going in, I received a letter from a woman named Reba, in Sweden, who had a young daughter with RP. She'd been trying to get Swedish agencies to help pay for a trip to our Center. Because we weren't "medical," she was denied financial aid. I told her if she could get over here, we would be happy to work with her daughter for free. It was the least I could do. If someone really wanted to take advantage of the program but didn't have the money, I couldn't sleep if I turned them down.

Reba's family and friends raised the necessary funds for the trip, so she and her daughter, Naomi, came over during the summer. Fortunately they had distant relatives living in the area, so housing was not an added expense. Naomi was a delightful nine-year-old who spoke perfect English. (I've always been amazed at how other countries educate their youth to speak more than one language. And English is usually their preferred second language.)

Before they came, Reba told me that she, herself, couldn't do much outside the home, because of her need to be available for her daughter. Sweden has long winter nights, when the sun peeks out for only a few hours even during midday, and Naomi, with her reduced vision, couldn't see well enough to walk the four blocks to her school. So her mother had to assist her in both directions.

We go along splendidly and Naomi responded favorably. After they returned to their home, I got a wonderful thank-you letter. Previously, Naomi's field of vision had been rapidly decreasing and she was regularly hurting herself, running into doorways, tables, and other objects. Reba reported that now Naomi was able to go to school by herself, even to participate in sports activities. No more bruises and injured limbs. Her ability to be mobile improved greatly. My heart was filled with joy for this young child and her mother.

Reba was pleased to find that her own life also improved. She was now able to join in the community around her and won a seat in the local government. Reba pledged to find a way to bring me over to Sweden, so I could start a Center like the one in Santa Rosa. I didn't hold my breath, but I was pleased she thought so highly of me and the work and wanted to share it with people in her homeland.

I wrote back, saying I would be more than happy to come if she could arrange it. I thought nothing more about it. The possibility of my traveling to Sweden seemed remote at best.

The program I stumbled upon was now helping others and I felt vindicated. Each time people completed a course at the Center, my determination was redoubled. In our first eighteen months, we worked with more than one hundred people who had serious eye problems. Clinical tests indicated that more than ninety percent showed improvement.

Working with the Center's participants was extremely rewarding. Memories of the time when I had such poor sight flooded back, as other people shared their experiences. I remembered when I thought there was no hope, that I would go completely blind. Back then, when I saw something beautiful, I tried to memorize every detail. I believed when my outer vision no longer functioned, I could call on my visual memory to provide me with pictures of beautiful things—images tucked away for a rainy, dark day.

One such image from about ten years before stands out in my mind. After talking most of the night, my sister Kathleen and I jumped in her van to go watch the sunrise from the top of a nearby mountain. I loved the flexibility of having a car. The freedom to drive away to watch the sun make its daily debut is a luxury that can hardly be fully appreciated until it's gone. Nor is it anything that can be provided by public transportation. And even if there was a bus out in the country, it wouldn't take me to the top of a mountain at dawn.

We arrived just in time. From our high vantage point, we saw the valley below, in a sea of thick grey fog. The peaks of the hills dotted the fog, as if they were miniature islands. Tall redwoods rose through it as well, promising hidden surprises underneath. The silence was mystical. The fog bank dulled all sounds.

Directly above our heads was the darkest blue-black sky, sparkling with millions of stars. Holding my breath, I turned toward the eastern horizon. In a line that only a master artist could have made was the most incredible blood-red gash, as if the sun had to tear the day open from the night.

From the blue-black above us to the scarlet horizon hugging the earth's edge were the most wonderful varying shades of blue—from the darkest to the faintest, almost pink where they touched the red scar. My breath was suspended for those few moments, as I waited for the sun to announce itself fully. Sunlight would disperse the fog, allowing the earth to be more visible. The gift of light, I knew, takes away shadows just as truth brings enlightenment.

The beauty the Universe provides cannot be matched by the greatest painter. I wanted desperately to capture the view, the colors, and especially the feeling of being in a holy place. I wished I was a photographer. Perhaps an artist of some kind. No, not even that, because if I didn't have sight, what good would pictures be? No, I wanted to be a writer. To paint pictures with words. That's what I wanted in order to preserve this magical, mystical morning.

As my attention returned to the present, I thought of my clients and their fears about losing their sight, and I was reminded that we all had another bond in common. No one wanted to lose the gift of seeing life's beautiful images. Smiles on babies' lips, tears of joy on a mother's face, a rose opening for sensual pleasures, or a sunset painting the sky. These events take place everywhere on the planet each day. They are the things people miss when they lose their ability to see. It's the beauty, not necessarily the function, we miss the most. As old memories fade, I continue to give thanks that I was able to regain my sight.

An unexpected champion came into my life. A woman named Eleanor called from the office of Willie Brown, one of the most powerful politicians in California. He was Speaker of the Assembly, wielding power with the best of them, one of the masters of the art of politics. I had not seen Assemblyman Brown in years.

I met him when I worked with Connections, the prisoner family organization. Family members of prisoners were not given much consideration by the prison staff, and that occasionally caused much grief to the family. Sometimes a prisoner was transferred to another prison and the family would not realize it until they came for a visit. On several occasions I remember having a nearly hysterical wife or mother in my office, wanting to know where her loved one was. The only State legislator who would help was Willie Brown. He never failed to get results from phone calls he made on our behalf. He carried weight, even back then. I had grown to respect him as a fair and concerned individual. He always kept his word and treated us with respect.

Over the years, I followed his rise to power in the State legislature through news reports. His home base was San Francisco, so my living near the city often gave me an opportunity to watch his smoke. He made enemies along the way, but always seemed to come out on top. I admired him back in the early Seventies and now admired him even more. He was legendary.

As I spoke to Eleanor on the phone, I assumed she had vision problems of some kind. She was very inquisitive, asking for documentation and literature to be sent to her at the office. I was happy to oblige.

She told me she was home with a flu bug one day and, for some reason, turned on the television set. Normally she was never home during the workweek and she could not remember the last time she watched daytime television. On that particular day, I was a guest on "People Are Talking." She felt as though fate had brought her attention to the show. She promised to call back after reviewing the literature I was to send.

A few weeks passed, and I had almost forgotten the call from Willie's assistant. Until Eleanor called again.

This time, she asked if I could come to her office. Without hesitation, I agreed. I liked going to San Francisco, and my sister Kellee was happy to drive with me into the city. When she was born, I had already left home, so working together gave us the chance to get closer and know one another better. Kellee was tall, almost six feet, and very attractive. Her youth and enthusiasm were contagious, and a little of her energy rubbed off on me at times. We had a great deal of fun together and welcomed any opportunity to get away from the office with one another.

I briefed Kellee on our way to the city. The meeting was set for two in the afternoon, so we got there early enough to find lunch and a parking place. Lunch is much easier to find than a parking space, believe me. San Francisco is a beautiful city, built on a small, hilly peninsula. Housing and parking are at a premium, though, and when we found a spot less than a block away from Willie's office; I counted it as our mini-miracle for the day!

We dressed like women executives on the off-chance we would run into Willie himself. I wanted us looking good. Kellee had a wonderful motto we had begun to live by. "It is better to look good than to feel good." It didn't always work, but we always made the attempt.

The receptionist told us we were expected and that the Speaker would be with us shortly. Now I was confused. What was going on? Was the appointment with Eleanor or with Willie?

Willie came out to greet us. Seeing him was wonderful. With introductions and small talk out of the way, he got right to the point. He always was a man who could cut to the heart of a situation, and now he was living up to his reputation. Basically, here was the story. He had an eye problem. It could be RP, though it affected his central sight more than one would expect with RP. His central sight was still functional, although reading was becoming more of a challenge. He wanted to know if I thought my program could help him. After recovering from the shock, I told him it would sure be worth trying. Since he was healthy and willing to work, I thought his chances of strengthening his eyes were good.

Once Willie makes up his mind, things move at the speed of light. He decided he would come to Santa Rosa and work with Kellee and me during his spring recess. Group work was not an option since, at the time, Willie wanted his involvement with me kept confidential. In politics, every weakness, real or imagined, would be exploited by his foes. We both understood. Fortunately, no groups were scheduled during the time he could make himself available. When something is meant to be, everything falls into place without effort. Obviously, this was one of those times.

I did not take the enormity of my responsibility lightly. I wanted to help Willie, not just for all the help he had given people in the past, but also because I respected him greatly. He was one of my heroes. It was also clear to me that if we were able to help him, he might be able to help us at the Center. Speaker Willie Brown was one of the most well-connected people I ever had the honor and privilege to meet. A lot was at stake in my taking him on as a client.

Kellee and I decided not to tell our coworkers. We told them to take off the week when Willie would be present. All the therapy except acupuncture would be done by the two of us. Kellee and I spent hours working out a schedule that would provide him with optimum therapy and training. We wanted the best possible results in as short a time as possible. Willie could give us only seven days. It was quite a challenge, and we had to make every day count.

◦❧◦

Willie, after being dropped off at our office, told his bodyguard/chauffeur to take the rest of the day off. It was a Sunday. Kellee and I waited nervously for his arrival.

He put us at ease immediately. After about an hour of introduction to the program, he suggested we go to brunch. He knew how to talk our language, Kellee's and mine. We took him to one of the best restaurants in Santa Rosa, called John Ash and Company. Unfortunately, most of the people in the know go to John Ash for Sunday brunch. Willie was recognized at once, and we were given the royal treatment. Kellee and I felt like celebrities. We giggled like schoolgirls at the thought of all the people wondering just who in the world we were, thinking we were important women to be dining out with the Speaker of the Assembly of the State of California. Tongues wagged busily that morning, let me tell you.

Willie was a most interesting conversationalist. There wasn't a subject or an opinion he didn't know or have. It was stimulating, and Kellee and I fell madly in love with him. Willie is married, as was Kellee, so romance wasn't what we were thinking about. He was just simply a powerful man and we loved his "presence." He was entertaining to boot. It was an irresistible combination.

During every day of our time together, we put in at least five to six hours of concentrated teaching and working. Willie was doing the eye exercises and the other disciplines in the program. As we got to know each other better, we all looked forward to the next day.

Lunchtime was always a treat and one afternoon Kellee and I decided to make a surprise excursion. The noon hour came rolling around and we told Willie we wanted to take him on a tour of the countryside in Santa Rosa. He was game for anything at this point!

We headed up to Howarith Park, a lovely lake on the east side of the city. Since school was in session, the area was nearly deserted when we arrived. We found a parking space in front of the lake. Still pretending to Willie that we were here for a quick look, Kellee popped open the trunk. She had picked up a gourmet picnic lunch from our neighborhood delicatessen—everything, including a red-and-white checkered tablecloth, cloth napkins, and real wine glasses.

Willie was totally surprised. We were thrilled at his response. We wanted to give something back to him for all of his sharing. By this time, we were good friends, close as a result of the experiences we went through together. We all, Kellee included, had faced the prospect of losing our sight. That bond is strong, as we knew from working with others. But we became closer to him than with anyone else in the past. Loving him was easy. His sense of humor, his kindness, and his caring made him even more attractive.

Willie was a funny man. In fact, so funny that Kellee and I were falling off the benches laughing so hard. He told us about the many political-rally picnics he attended in the past. He couldn't remember how many pieces of fried chicken now, how many bites of potato salad he downed in his long career. And before he could eat, he usually had to give a speech. This, he said, was the first picnic he had been to in over twenty years where he didn't have to give a talk before he was able to eat.

Just as he was finishing his narration, about ten large geese came waddling over, trying to get some leftover lunch. I told Willie that his constituents heard he was there and were coming over for a speech. We were hysterical by this time. The squawking birds surrounded Willie as if he were a goose-magnet. I'm not going to say Willie was scared, but I could see he was a bit nervous. When he tried feeding a sliced tomato (still on his fork) to the biggest of the bunch, he found out how nasty those birds can get. The leader of the pack refused to eat it! We were collapsing with laughter watching one of the most powerful politicians in California using a fork as he tried to force-feed a reluctant, angry goose.

In a hug, Willie turned on the offensive. "I'll make pâté out of you in a second if you don't stop hissing at me," he growled. Kellee and I couldn't stop laughing and were absolutely no help to him at all. He was such a good sport, though, that the geese eventually got some very tasty morsels. His battles in the political arena had taught him well. At that point, I was certain there was nothing Willie couldn't do if he put his mind to it. I'm sure many a governor found that out when coming up against him in a political fight. He was and is a tough customer. To us on that wonderful spring day, though, he was a love. We laughed at him and with him.

We had a special time with Willie. There were no hidden agendas, no political fires to tend, and I think Willie had as good a time as we did. However, the reason he was there was not to have a mini-vacation, but to get somewhere with his vision. We worked hard and we played hard. Who says you can't have a good time getting healthy?

Our final day came all too quickly. I was sad to see Willie go. He was one of the most challenging and interesting people I ever worked with. The experience was educational for me, and I'm sure it was for him, as well. To mark the day, we went to another of the finer restaurants in Santa Rosa. It had become a tradition that when the course was over, we celebrated by having a party or going to lunch. This was no exception.

We were toasting one another, all three of us. Suddenly, Willie put his wine glass down and asked Kellee if she was wearing blue mascara. Confused by the question and not realizing its significance at first, she acknowledged that she was. However, I was completely excited, as I realized the importance of what just happened. Willie's central sight was improving!

He was astonished and started looking around, suddenly much more aware of his ability to see clearly. Though he had not lost a great deal of sight when he came to the Center, he did notice increasing difficulty seeing people's eyes clearly, especially at a medium distance. Since a good politician depends on his ability to "read" people, especially his opponents, this put him at a disadvantage and he wanted to improve his vision as soon as possible.

His discovery that day at lunch was joyous for us all. And what a relief! We'd pushed hard over those seven days and Willie definitely improved. I wanted more than anything for him to notice a difference and now I felt like a ton of bricks had been lifted off my shoulders. Willie wasn't the type of person to be fooled, or to fool himself. His astute sense of what was going on with his eyes, and his quick mind, showed him the improvement was a reality. If he noticed a difference, then it was there.

He asked what we needed to further our work. Our answer was direct and to the point. Money. Funds would allow us to get the necessary research done. In that way the program could be fully evaluated. It also would help us keep the doors open. Willie said he'd do what he could. That's all I needed to hear. I knew the Universe had taken a strong step in getting my program off the exploratory level and into the mainstream.

Willie left for Sacramento—back to the mill, so to speak. We were flattered and excited when he later invited Kellee and me to one of his renowned fund-raising parties. Willie Brown had a reputation for putting on fabulous parties, and we accepted with a breathless yes.

Wow! What were we going to wear? Kellee and I looked at each other and said simultaneously, "Time to go shopping!" Usually a broken shoelace gave us a good excuse to go shopping. But with an invitation to a party of this caliber, we really had a reason to get ourselves to the nearest mall.

Kellee found the most beautiful, slinky, peacock-blue silk dress. I had my black-and-white number, so we were all set. The rhinestone earrings cost us over sixty bucks, but they were worth it. They added such class to Kellee's dress. I found a stunning little black cocktail hat with netting to top it all off. Kellee was also going to wear stiletto high heels, putting her over the six-foot mark. I had to admit, even though she was my sister, that she would be the most strikingly attractive woman at the party. Me? I looked like a white gospel singer in a long robe. Fashions for big women had come a long way, but still had an even longer way to go. I did the best I could.

Arriving at the hall for the party, I walked into a crowd of party-goers who looked like they belonged on the set of "Dynasty." Elegant tuxedos and long beautiful gowns were on parade. A quartet of musicians played classical music as people lingered in front of the mini-bars sprinkled around the room. This was a high-class event, that's for sure.

It was a five-hundred-dollar-a-plate fund-raising dinner. Kellee and I had been invited free, and the people at our table had been hand-selected by Willie personally. I almost fainted as I was introduced to the guests sitting with us. A vice-president of Blue Cross on one side and the president of the California Optometric Association on the other. Willie told us he always arranges the place cards himself. He certainly was the master at getting the right people to meet at the right time and place. His ability to "network" went way beyond anything I ever encountered.

It was all going too fast for me. In fact, it unnerved me completely. I wasn't good at lobbying. My exposure to this high level of power-brokers was between nothing and zero. With the shock of the possibilities, in combination with drinking on an empty stomach, I was a total failure. I didn't make the connections Willie had envisioned my making. I know it was a disappointment to him, but more to the point, I was crushed. I was given the chance of a lifetime, and I blew it.

Kellee, on the other hand, was a big hit. She danced until the wee hours of the morning and had an absolute ball. I could only lie back in the car seat on the way home, trying not to throw up again, and pray the gods would give me another chance at the brass ring. Kellee laughed her head off the entire way. If she hadn't been my best friend and my sister, I would have hated her.

Sure, Kellee could laugh at my terrible hangover and depression the following day. She hadn't blown it like I had. But I knew what I wouldn't do next time. I sure wouldn't have a drink when I was in that kind of company.

Thankfully, a new class was starting. It would keep me busy and prevent me from dwelling on my personal failure to work the party. Helping people with their vision problems was what I did best. They didn't care if I couldn't make it in the big time, mingling with the hotshots. As long as I could help them, I was a success. Getting over my party-trauma took quite a while, though.

⊚☙

In the meantime, a trip to Jacksonville, Illinois, was coming up. A teacher at the Illinois School for the Deaf contacted me after reading about our program in a magazine. She worked with children who, along with being deaf, had the additional tragic problem of losing their sight. It is a condition known as Usher's Syndrome, one of the different types of retinitis pigmentosa.

I had lain awake thinking about what being blind and deaf might be like. My eyes filled with tears as I thought of those youngsters and their difficulties at communicating. My heart hurt for them, and I vowed that if I could do anything to help them, I would move heaven and earth to do it.

My tickets were bought, my bags were packed. I was leaving to talk to the parents and staff of the school. The sting of my failure at the party faded as I left the Bay Area and headed to the Deaf School in Illinois. Work is a great healer to the psyche.

14

CAN'T HEAR THE MUSIC CAN'T SEE THE LIGHT

The driveway curved toward a formidable monster of a building housing the School for the Deaf. The trees lining the drive were barren, creating a spider-web silhouette against the grey, overcast sky. Winter wasn't quite gone, nor had spring quite arrived. The snow that hid the dead-looking lawn had melted, leaving lifeless blades of grass visible to all who passed by.

The building that dominated the driveway was over a hundred and fifty years old. It contained administrative offices and guest quarters. Newer, more comfortable buildings behind that massive stone and brick structure housed the children. I had no preconceptions of what a school for the deaf would be like, but I was taken aback by the coldness of the main building. I was relieved to find the children and young adults living in a more modern and homey environment.

The old building, however, was where I would spend the two nights of my stay. My room, on the second floor, was large and had a bleak, empty, institutional feeling. It had six twin beds, three on each side, and seemed to hold troubling memories of the time it housed the deaf children. My occupying only one small bed made the emptiness all the more evident.

If that building held grim feelings from its past, at least the people at the school were friendly. I was introduced to several teachers and members of the administration, then spent the remainder of the first day getting familiar with things.

At lunchtime, my guide and I headed for the main dining room. The first thing I noticed was the silence: not many voices, but a tremendous amount of activity, as people were talking, even laughing— with their hands. This was the special world of the deaf. I was overwhelmed by this environment, so different from the one I was accustomed to, and I felt like a real outsider.

I began to take a closer look at these young people. Their ages ranged from six to around the late teens, maybe early twenties. My guide, a woman, told me a great many of the children lost their hearing from measles. I was dumbfounded. I saw no excuse for this preventable tragedy.

Not everyone was deaf from a childhood disease, though. Eight children at the school had been diagnosed as having Usher's Syndrome, the deaf and sight-loss disease. I would be seeing some of them and meeting their parents the next day.

I was asked to make a formal presentation about my program, which parents and teachers would attend. The school also invited members of the press. It was going to be a big day, and with all the new experiences awaiting me, I hoped I would be ready. This was much different from what I was used to dealing with, and my self-confidence was between shaky and nonexistent. Could I offer these children any hope?

Usher's was not totally unfamiliar to me. In the past, I worked with several people who had Usher's Syndrome, and they responded favorably to the program. They were all adults, though, by the time they'd come to me. These were children, which made me especially aware of the awesome responsibility an adult had toward a child. It can be overwhelming. In no way did I want to give anyone false hope or mislead any child's parents. I could easily put myself in their place. Maybe that was even part of the problem growing like a weed inside me. I felt their pain, their anguish for their children. If our places were reversed, I know I'd have moved heaven and earth to help a child of mine function better in the world. This experience wasn't going to be easy, and I knew that. I prayed for help and guidance.

Lunch was over and the time came to take a stroll around the grounds. Walking across the yard toward the building that housed the classrooms, I noticed a young girl standing on the steps. She was a beautiful child, with dark curly hair framing her face, and looked to be around ten years old. She was wearing a pair of thick glasses, making her dark eyes look huge. For some unknown reason, my own eyes started to tear up. She and I made a strong connection, looking at one another, a connection I couldn't explain. She stared at me, and I couldn't break the eye contact. I felt, at a very deep level, that she and I knew one another. There definitely was a bond, an extremely strong bond. I asked my guide who this young girl was.

"Oh, that's Tanya, one of the children with Usher's. You'll meet her parents tomorrow."

When she heard my sharp intake of breath, she asked if I was all right. All right? Sure. But I began to feel I was here for a special reason, even though I didn't know what it was.

My heart was pounding as we entered the school. I'd never had such a physical reaction to meeting another human being—ever. It was as if there were strings, invisible strings, attached to that child, pulling me closer to her. Internally I was reeling with the impact of that encounter. Without words, I had connected to this child. Was she the reason I came? Suddenly I wondered: could she be my daughter? The possibility was stunning, overwhelming, yet when I looked again, I realized she was much younger than my daughter would be. The yearning to find my child was not to be satisfied on that day.

As we approached the classroom, my guide said I was in for another surprise. She began to tell me of a different little girl, also—to my surprise—named Tanya. The other Tanya was giving the teachers a challenge. She was a little younger than the child I had just seen, and some of the teachers thought she might be mentally retarded. How odd, I thought, finding two Tanyas, both suffering from the same genetic defect in the same school. I was beginning to think this was a special trip in more than one way. It was as if I had stepped into the Twilight Zone.

Tanya number two was a small, shy, black child. As I looked on, the instructor was attempting to teach her how to say "dog" in sign language. The instructor would raise a picture of a dog and signal Tanya to tell her what the picture was. I saw Tanya looking, moving her head side to side, up and down, in a way that only people with a very limited field of vision tend to do. After she had fully examined the picture, Tanya started to snap the fingers of her right hand.

The teacher asked her again to sign what the picture was, and Tanya repeated the gesture, snapping her fingers. I saw the frustration on the teacher's face. Since I didn't know sign language, I asked my guide to show me the sign for dog. She snapped her fingers, about ear high, and then with the same hand, patted the side of her thigh.

It hit me like a bolt of lightning. Of course! When the teacher finished snapping and did the second part of the sign, her hand left Tanya's limited field of sight. Tanya didn't know it was a two-part sign. The teacher was well-educated in regard to the deaf but didn't fully understand the limitation that a restricted visual field put on Tanya's learning potential.

My mind was reeling. Could this be the reason they thought Tanya was mentally retarded? Because she was slow in learning and didn't seem to get the "picture"? It was obvious to me that the teachers needed a quick course in eye disease such as retinitis pigmentosa. With better understanding, they could be certain their teaching methods included the special needs of children who were visually impaired and who had hearing loss.

I noticed closed-circuit television equipment in the room. As a result of my own experience of limited vision, I immediately suggested they put their hand-signing instructions on video. With a smaller screen, they could show Tanya the entire sign.

That worked like a charm. I could see Tanya's face light up with recognition and understanding. She had become as frustrated as the teachers, probably beginning to think—as they did already— that she was stupid and retarded. Finally, someone recognized her problem! No wonder she was so shy and retreating. My heart was breaking for both Tanyas who were trying to live in a world that didn't quite understand them. Having the problem myself gave me the ability to see more clearly what was going on. As it turned out, Tanya was a very bright child.

❦

That evening, when I was alone on the second floor of the ancient building, my mind couldn't stop thinking about the two Tanyas. Both demonstrated a strong spirit and presence. Both entered my heart, never to leave again. I wept for all the children who had to suffer and for fear I wouldn't be able to do much for them. I loved them immediately and prayed that somehow they would be helped.

Falling asleep was difficult. The building held noises of its own, moaning and groaning. My sleep was fitful and I had terrifying dreams. Images of silent screams from rooms along the narrow hallways, lit by one bare bulb every hundred feet, kept me restless. The ghosts of children who were left by saddened, heavy-hearted parents wandered those hallways. This old building had a history of over a hundred years, and not always happy years.

Just by its nature, this had not been the most nurturing, loving environment for children to grow up in. I'm sure people tried their best, but I know it left scars. In my sleep, vulnerable to the energy that prowls the night, I learned more than a hearing person usually does about the world of the deaf. I was glad when the sun appeared, to chase away the ghosts of the past.

⟨✦⟩

The meeting with the parents and staff went well. I explained what my program involved and what they should expect from it. They asked questions that were well thought-out and I was pleased with their response to my presentation.

Afterward, the parents of children with Usher's met with me privately. We discussed the possibility of a trip to our Center. We talked about the financial aspects of bringing instructors, interpreters, and parents. It would be a costly venture. I told them the Center would reduce or waive its fees, however we did need to raise funds for transportation and housing. The group decided to begin a fund-raising drive; I agreed to do the same in California. My heart was filled with compassion for the parents and their children. If the program helped prevent their kid from losing their sight, and therefore their ability to communicate, we would do it even if it was free. Of course, I was committing the entire staff of the Center, but I felt they would, if necessary, donate their time to these special children.

Arriving back home was a relief. The trip had been difficult emotionally and I felt completely drained. My staff and Board of Directors agreed with the plan. We started to prepare a summer class for the young people from the Deaf School.

∽❦∾

Things were beginning to fall into place at the Center. The best news was that we were apparently going to receive a $100,000 grant from the California Department of Rehabilitation, a State agency. The application we submitted had been tentatively approved. Now we had to take it the rest of the way through the maze of committees and hoops that a nonprofit organization must jump through.

The grant would be the answer to my prayers. It, together with the money from our general fund-raising, would allow us to expand our services and begin gathering the documentation necessary for acceptance in the medical community.

∽❦∾

Nine of the children from the Deaf School, their mothers, and two teachers were scheduled to attend a two-week program in late June 1985. We wanted to be certain we were prepared to provide everything they needed.

At one point, we decided to have a dance and sell tickets for it. Kellee, who had become my right hand, was ready to help get the event kicked off so we could raise money for the children's two-week stay.

Through Willie Brown's assistant, we got introductions to people in high places. We managed to get free airline tickets for the kids and their families to fly to Disneyland after the program was complete. Hotels in the area were willing to give major discounts. Everyone seemed to be pulling together, and it was a learning process for us all.

We'd never put together a fund-raising drive before, so the process was a real eye-opener. It had a certain life of its own, thrilling in many ways, as we were touching members of the community and getting them excited about our work with the children. People were receptive and willing to help.

⚜

Ru was thirteen. So far, so good. The early stage of his teenage life was going well. We were getting along okay. He was proud of what I was doing and loved being in the limelight. He was not inhibited at all by being on television, whether it was local or national. His confidence and ability to communicate allowed me to feel I was doing an adequate job of being a mother.

He was turning out to be a wonderful human being in spite of my neuroses. All the moves from place to place apparently hadn't hurt him; instead they had made him flexible in adapting to new situations. He was still the light of my life. There was no one else in the entire world to whom I could talk so honestly.

My administrative duties were nearly killing me. My blood pressure was up and I was having difficulty sleeping. I hated being in charge of everything and found I definitely didn't have what it takes to be a good manager. Eleven people were now working with me at the Center, and we had eight outside, independent directors. I decided to notify the Board of Directors that I wanted to be in charge of clinical work and research, and no more. I requested they find another person to be Executive Director. My skills and talents did not lie in bookkeeping, personnel management, and other office duties. I wanted to work with the people who came to us for help. That's where my talent was, not to mention my heart. I tried being an executive type, but it just wasn't for me. Things were getting backed up and I didn't even know where to look for the problems, much less the solutions. I wanted to hand over the reins to someone more qualified than I was. It had been my baby, but the baby was growing up, and I couldn't meet its needs anymore.

When the deaf children landed at the airport in San Francisco, we had quite a reception for them. Their arrival became a media event. Television crews from most of the local news stations were waiting for the group to come down the jet-way. We had a few dozen colorful balloons so the children and their guardians would be able to identify us as soon as they came into the terminal. This trip had taken five months, working some fifteen to twenty hours a week, for us to plan and organize. We were exhausted, but happy the day finally arrived.

Being busy was good, because it kept my doubts and fears at bay. I usually said several prayers a day to ask for help for these children. Now, as I waited for them, such special kids, to make their entrance into the waiting area, my heart was pounding and all my self-doubts came flooding in with a vengeance. What if we couldn't help them? How would they take it? How would I take it? What would the press do? Well, it was too late to stop at this point, so onward and upward. I took a deep breath and smiled at everyone around me.

Trust me. You can't learn sign language in a few weeks, and especially not just from flash cards. All I succeeded in doing with my version of signing was to confuse the kids. They handled the problem with wonderful directness. They requested that I sit on my hands.

One of the teachers from the school in Illinois became the official translator. It was slow going, but her presence was a blessing. Otherwise, I don't think we could have completed the sessions at all, much less had any degree of success.

The children were wonderful. There was one family of three boys, ranging in age from eleven to nineteen. The youngest, Will, was particularly endearing. He had some speech and, thanks to two huge amplifying devices, partial hearing. He could communicate pretty well. Then there were the two Tanyas. The older Tanya, with lovely brown hair, was the one I first saw at the school that dreary February day in Illinois. It was she, of course, with whom I bonded so strongly in our first instant of eye contact. She was shy, but apparently not afraid of anything. Her eagerness to get on with the program was truly inspiring. Her goal, her mother told me, was to get rid of those thick glasses. I kept my fingers crossed mentally.

The other Tanya, the youngest of the group, was also the shyest and most timid. She was a beautiful child, with hair in sweet braids tied at the ends by colorful ribbons. Her mother was able to be there, and I know it was a special time for the two of them. We all got along with love, laughter, and some tears.

Tanya's limited field of vision had impaired her educational progress (she's the child they thought was retarded). In order to communicate with her, one had to sign about twelve to fourteen inches away, directly in front of her face. If a person were not within her field of view, she couldn't tell what was happening. But since we knew her special needs, we designed the program to meet them.

⧉

The two weeks were full with activity. The work was incredibly challenging and often very frustrating. My desire to communicate with the children burned strongly. But I was dependent on the interpreter, and given the delay between my words and her signing, my stories needed to be short and my instructions to the point.

In spite of the difficulties, we began to be a close-knit group. Hugs all the time, not just upon arrival and departure, became the norm. Loving them all was easy. My fears melted as I saw how they progressed. The exercises were a snap for them. They caught on quickly and loved to do them. The days were passing all too swiftly.

My dear friend Elliot Kaplan volunteered to give the children their "before and after" eye exams. He was excited to hear about their progress and looked forward to retesting them on their last day. I knew changes were taking place, but the icing on the cake would be when clinical tests confirmed my intuition and observations.

Little Tanya—the child who had been considered retarded because of her inability to learn the deaf sign for dog; who was shy, timid, and unable to communicate with people unless they were a few inches away—came out of her shell. She was laughing and interacting enthusiastically with the other children, even from across the room! I knew her field of vision was much better. Her enhanced ability to function, communicate, and even feel secure within herself was obvious to us all. She had transformed into a most beautiful preteen butterfly. My heart was full when I looked at her smiling face. No longer shy and scared, she was full of ginger and spice.

Will, the child who heard with the help of two large amplifying devices, fantasized that he would come back and work with us after he graduated from high school. He liked acupuncture and wasn't afraid of the needles at all. He even asked if he could take some home to do it on himself. We all laughed at his bold concept of self-help acupuncture.

❧

The last day came all too fast. The staff really became attached to these wonderful children. I was gratified we had done well and knew I would miss them terribly.

Elliot showed up as scheduled and began his testing. Each child's parent and both teachers were able to sit in on the examination. Elliot was happy to answer any questions they had. He was so patient and wanted them to know exactly what his findings were.

My Tanya with the thick glasses came out of Elliot's office wearing a huge grin. Her eyes tested better without the glasses, and she had taken them off. She didn't need them anymore! Tears of joy fell down more than one person's cheek that afternoon. The visual function of every child had improved. We had no failure that session. A one-hundred-percent success rate! Let me tell you, the celebration and party that took place that afternoon and evening couldn't be topped. The experience will live forever in my heart.

The children had been taught how to work on their own when they returned to their homes and school. The techniques and training would allow them to continue helping themselves to maintain healthier eyes. They had achieved a great deal in those two short weeks.

I was pleased that the teachers from the school were able to attend as well—not just because they translated for us, but also because of their learning the discipline themselves. In the future, if more children suffered the double whammy of deafness and vision loss, the teachers would be able to start them on the program at the school. I was very proud of our work that summer.

We took a financial loss however. The Center was now in the red. Ironically, we were able to help people improve their sight, even in the face of great odds. Yet, we weren't doing well monetarily. Thank goodness the grant we applied for had been approved. We were in the last stages of completing the forms so we could start receiving that income.

We were counting on it to pull us out of the financial hole we had sunk into.

Then the media got wind of a political scandal. Apparently, members of the medical committees didn't approve of a nonmedical center getting funded. After all, retinitis pigmentosa was classified as a non-treatable, non-curable eye disease. Who were we to be claiming improvement? Various foes of Assemblyman Brown came out of their corners swinging, not reluctant to throw some low punches. My picture was placed next to Willie Brown's in a large newspaper, the Sacramento Bee, in a story that blew the grant out of proportion. Our Center had become a pawn on the chessboard of political gamesmanship.

The issues, I realized, didn't really involve us or what we did. We were caught in a larger, more far-reaching process of political intrigue, of ambitions, fears, favors, and alliances. The whole matter was entirely out of our hands. What could I say or do? I had screwed up a friendly networking party that Willie made available to me. Did I think I was going to be able to compete here, in the cutthroat world of high-roller politics? I hated like hell not being able to fight back somehow. But too much was at stake, and neither I nor the Center had the financial resources to wait the situation out.

The money from the grant would have pulled us out of the red and allowed us to document our results in a much more precise way. It would have lasted a year, and with that funding approved, we'd have been able to approach private foundations for money for additional projects. If the grant was delayed, however, we wouldn't survive the fall of 1985. Political and media sharks smelled blood. A feeding frenzy ensued and we, unfortunately, were the dinner.

Politics is a dirty business. We became the victims of other people's prejudices and ignorance. The funds were held up in committee. Our contact told us word had come down the grapevine that "hell would freeze" before funds were released to our organization.

I gave up. I just couldn't keep going in the hole every day to make the place work. It was too much.

Telling everyone the Center was folding was so hard for me. Many people had relocated to be able to work with us. I felt I failed them personally. Everyone was sad and, perhaps, in some way they blamed me. My feelings were all over the map. Angry, frustrated, and most of all, guilty—believing I had personally failed. My attempt at jousting with windmills had been a flop.

So the Center closed its doors for good. A few months passed before I was able to regroup, and I decided to continue the work on my own. I had been invited to do a program in England. And my friend Reba, in Sweden, had worked hard to arrange speaking engagements for me in her homeland. I decided to spread out and work overseas for a while. My plea to heaven was to be able to do the work, and I was willing to go anywhere to accomplish that goal! If America (or at least California) didn't want me, I would go elsewhere, anywhere I was wanted.

Though I was not a good director for the Center, my plan for improving and maintaining vision was sound. It worked. My inability to run a large organization led me into failure. I had to learn that lesson and move on. Instead of taking on any more responsibility for a large group, I decided to go solo, running a very small overhead—just me!

15

WHAT'S A DRACHMA

When the door closes, another always opens. Since the doors to my dream, the Center for Eye Health Education, had closed, I was curious as to what life would offer, what new road I would embark upon. The Center's closing was a real blow to my self-confidence and I couldn't easily let go of feelings of guilt and failure. A new project would help chase those blues away.

Reba had been working on setting up speaking engagements for me in Sweden. Simultaneously, another friend was able to put together a large class for me to teach in London. Things were looking up. Reba also had a surprise waiting for me in Sweden. Not only did she start an organization dedicated to teaching my methods, but she also made contact with the European Retinitis Pigmentosa Foundation. This organization, with thousands of members all over the world, was having its annual convention in Germany in May 1986, the time I was scheduled to be in Sweden. I don't know how she did it, but Reba was able to get me an invitation to speak at their Conference.

That Conference was to be a three-day affair. Half the audience would be eye doctors and scientists doing research. The other half would be people with RP, or friends and family of RP sufferers. Over 700 were planning to attend. I was flabbergasted but terribly excited about the opportunity for that kind of exposure. My dream of having a serious study of my program conducted grew back to a full-blown possibility. If it could be done at all, this would be the place to get the interest stimulated.

Ru stayed in the States for this trip. He was in school, a teenager. He also had a girlfriend and travel with Mom wasn't on his agenda. With mixed emotions, I let him stay with Kathleen for the duration. I made our travel arrangements to Europe.

My sister Kellee and I arrived in London twelve days before the British class began. I was also invited to speak at the Swiss Touch for Health Convention, in Geneva. My ego was inflating with the flurry of acknowledgment from my European contacts. It certainly was taking the sting out of my recent business failure at the Center.

The weather was cold and overcast, with wind streaming down from the North Sea. It chilled us to the bone, even through layers of sweaters and coats, but neither of us had been overseas as adults, so we explored London despite being frozen to the core.

It is certainly one of the most lively and exciting cities in the world. Its smells, sights, and sounds are as varied as the people that make up its population. History greeted us on every street corner. I could imagine seeing chimney sweeps hopping from the rooftops in a scene out of the movie Mary Poppins. I thought I could hear the hoof beats of the Household Cavalry, escorting the Queen's carriage as she paraded through the city. As much as we loved London, however, its cold temperature was getting to us. We went to the travel agent the very next day to see about the soonest possible transportation to the Swiss Alps, where the convention would be held the following weekend. We rashly decided that at least Switzerland, snow and all, couldn't possibly be any colder than this freezing island.

We went to the largest travel agency in England. The woman we worked with was fantastic. She obviously enjoyed helping us, though probably regarded us as silly Americans. At one point, I caught her smiling at us sort of secretly. After all, we were really being idiots—having a great time with our childlike enthusiasm and playing "what if?" with these exciting and exotic destinations.

Traveling and staying in Switzerland, we realized, would be outrageously expensive. We were in shock. The travel agent was optimistic about getting us a vacation somewhere, however.

Since Switzerland was out, she asked where else we were interested in going for a vacation.

Kellee and I looked at one another and both said about the same thing: "Something cheap and in the sun." We sounded like clones. Without batting an eyelash, the agent started playing with the keys on her computer terminal.

"What about the Canary Islands?"

Sounded find to us, but we had to investigate what the exchange rate would be. We learned early in our travel that changing money more than once makes the banks rich. We lost too much on those transactions. We also wanted to go where the U.S. dollar was the strongest.

The money exchange was in the basement. While I kept our place in line, Kellee ran down a circular stairway and got in the shortest line to learn the current exchange rate of each new destination we considered. Then she hurried back up the stairs so we could consult.

After figuring the angles, we decided the Canary Islands were too rich for our blood. Seems it's the playground of the rich Saudis. Back to the computer oracle. What about the south of Spain?

Back down the spiraling staircase for Kellee, as she barely had time to catch her breath.

Nope. Spain was out too.

Finally, the woman said, as if this was the bottom of the bargain travel barrel, "What about Greece?"

When Kellee learned what Greek money was called and got ready to race down the stairs again, I think she finally cracked under the physical strain. I was afraid she would collapse in a breathless heap right on the floor.

"What the hell is a drachma?" she pleaded. I felt she was close to hysteria.

Before long we found out exactly what a drachma was. It was money that meant we could go to Greece for a week, stay at a nice hotel, eat at least three meals a day, and have something left over for tourist-type activities. This was our kind of vacation spot. The dollar went far in Greece. The drachma and Greece were right up our financial alley.

"Book it," we said. We got tickets on a flight leaving the next day. We hadn't been in London more than thirty-six hours and were getting ready to leave.

We didn't consider until we were on the plane and halfway to Greece that this might not be a good thing for two single American women to do. We were headed to a place where terrorists regroup and are accepted as part of the population. But choosing to ignore our fear, we continued on the flight with excitement. Except when a snobby English woman turned to us from her seat and said we should be very careful. She warned us that the Greeks hated Americans. She advised that we tell anyone who asked that we were Canadians.

Kellee and I began to think about staying on the plane and going right back to England. A real round-trip. Then a nice-looking middle-aged man who overheard the woman warning us about Greece introduced himself as a native of Greece and told us he would personally see to it that we enjoyed our stay there. As we were easing out of our growing fear, the woman turned to us again and said, "Beware of Greeks bearing gifts." I think she was just jealous.

The Athens airport was pure pandemonium. We learned later that a TWA plane had been bombed on its way to Athens an hour before our flight landed. Thank goodness for our newfound friend. He helped us get a taxi and took us to a decent hotel in downtown Athens with a view of the Acropolis. Everything was breathtaking and mind-blowing all at the same time.

Over eight million people lived in Athens. They all seemed to drive cars and their cars all seemed to have the horn stuck on full blast. In ways, it reminded me of some older cities I had visited in Mexico. Dirty, busy, noisy, polluted from car exhaust and diesel emissions. And old…old all around.

Plus, the language was a problem. It sounded like no language I'd heard in my whole life. I don't think I could ever understand Greek.

With assurances that we would be safe, our host and volunteer travel-guide bade us goodnight. He and Kellee had talked horses and he made plans to show us his ranch the following day. We agree to meet him early the next morning.

Kellee found a Swedish soccer team. Or, more accurately, they found Kellee and were soon dancing the night away at the disco on the roof of our hotel. I bowed out early, as I was still suffering from jet lag. Besides, loud music and dark rooms were not my cup of tea. The last time I went out in the evening to hear music, I was listening to songs I loved to dance to when a stranger, a man in the night club, came over and asked me to dance. After I got over the surprise, I joyfully said sure and followed him onto the dance floor. Unfortunately, since the room was so dark, I never found him in the crowd. After standing for a few moments in confusion, trying to determine if I had a dance partner, I finally gave up and fumbled my way back to the table. I never found him. I worried all night that he was "Mr. Right" and I couldn't see in the dark well enough to hold onto him. Maybe that's why I was alone. But maybe not, either.

I wanted to fall asleep, but sleep was not to come. This city of millions on a warm, balmy night was just not quiet enough to allow it. It was as if every household had its windows open wide to lure the breeze inside, which meant all the sounds that ordinarily would be kept inside—loud televisions, blasting stereos, raucous family squabbles—were now escaping to the outside. All this added to the usual city of noises traffic and never-ending nightlife. The streets, old and curved, carried the noise as if it were river water, eddying and whirling into every possible crack and crevice. My ears, supersensitive to the language and environment due to culture shock, caught every sound. This was getting tiresome, and I was beginning to show signs of fatigue and stress from sleep deprivation. I'd not had a good night's sleep since leaving California.

By morning I was desperate. This wasn't my idea of a vacation. I wanted peace, quiet, and sunny beaches. Not noise from tens of millions of people competing for my attention while I was trying to sleep. My mind was made up. I would ask our friend to recommend a quiet place we might go to. Kellee agreed. Just mention sunshine and beaches to her, and she's got her tanning oil all ready.

Our friend was completely understanding and, after two phone calls at the front desk, had our dream vacation all arranged.

This first call was to his sister, who had a room open at her small hotel, which overlooked the Mediterranean on the island of Crete. The second was to the domestic airline. He booked two seats for us at midnight, on the last plane to leave Athens for Crete.

This was an internal domestic flight and security was not as tight as it was on international flights. We did not go through metal detectors or have our personal belongings x-rayed. That felt odd, since a bomb had exploded on another flight to Athens that same weekend.

Kellee and I agreed not to talk loudly or make it obvious that we were Americans. As we settled down in the waiting area to kill time until the flight left, I picked up a newspaper lying beside me and pretended to read.

Moments later, I saw a bright flash. (God, was it terrorists?) I looked up to see Kellee standing in front of me laughing her head off, camera in hand.

"What are you doing?" I whispered urgently.

Kellee was cracking up. She pointed to me and said, "You idiot, you were reading the paper upside down."

I didn't think it was funny. I was trying to be inconspicuous and my insensitive, unaware, crazy sister had just signed our death warrants, or at least notified every terrorist in the building that we were Americans on the loose.

Then I saw the humor in it and started laughing myself. Pretty soon the entire waiting room, so full that people were sitting on the floor, was laughing with us. Not that they understood the reason for the laughter; it was just contagious. I think tensions had been high since the earlier plane was bombed. Our laughter was a release for all of us.

So much for going quietly through life. Oh well, if we were going to be kidnapped as hostages or shot for being Americans, at least we'd have fun on the way out. We decided then and there that rather than being afraid, we'd be ourselves. I think, in the long run, that made our adventures even more fun and exciting. Fear is such a crippler. Having no night vision and still being visually impaired despite my improved sight added enough anxiety to my life. I'd be damned if I was going to let the possibility of a terrorist attack interfere with my life. I recognized clearly that if I postponed a trip or didn't do something due to fear of terrorism, the terrorist had won without even trying.

We were happy with our new attitude. Until we saw the airport guards in Crete carrying Uzis. Not a good sign. But it was midnight and we were too tired to get hysterical, so we hopped in a taxi, gave the driver the address our friend had written down, and set out to find our lodging for the next week. Our destination was a little fishing village called Agios Nicholas. Home away from home for the next seven days.

We arrived long after midnight and the taxi dumped us on the doorstep, leaving us alone in the quiet night. Should we wake the people up? We saw no signs, nor were any lights on. Oh dear. What do we do now?

Just as we were about to knock, the door opened and a beautiful older woman with black hair pulled back off her face welcomed us in. In halting English, she said we could take care of everything in the morning. For now, since it was so late and we were obviously tired, we should go right to our room. "Just go to sleep and I'll see you in the morning." As we struggled up three flights of steep and winding stairs, we were too weary to think. Throwing our luggage in a corner, we chose our beds and collapsed in a heap.

When I woke up, the sun was shining in; Kellee was already lying on the balcony, working on her tan. Our room, we discovered, was the entire third floor. It was huge, and the balcony was almost as large, running the entire length of the building. Our view included the harbor, the sea, and the little village that clustered around the inlet. This was perfect! Our luck was holding on the good side, that's for sure.

❧

Legend says Zeus was born on Crete. Legends usually have some truth in them somewhere, and if there was a god named Zeus, I could believe he had been born on this magical and timeless island.

We heard that the ruins of an ancient city lay nearby, a city that existed in 1500 B.C. We took a taxi there, and I was amazed to see magnificent ancient structures of stone still standing, showing clearly how the city had been laid out.

At the palace, I took off my sandals and placed my bare feet on the smooth, warm steps. It was so peaceful, so quiet, that I began to meditate. I started to see glimpses of scenes from an old movie. Or at least that's what I thought at first. I saw people standing in the courtyard and, on either side, large flames, huge torches. The glimpse lasted only a few seconds. I called for Kellee to come over and started telling her about my "vision."

To our astonishment, Kellee pointed out some large flat stones alongside the stairs in which scooped-out hollow areas still bore the marks of fire. Could they have been torch-lamps centuries ago? Did the rocks hold memories? Had the images pouring into my consciousness somehow shown me how people lived so long ago? Of course, I realized that the fires could just as well have burned there a month ago or the previous day, but still it was a startling revelation, my first experience of seeming to absorb the energy of a place and then have visions of that kind. Whatever was going on, it had been jarring.

Also, I was excited about the possibility of its happening again. The Greeks have had a working civilization for a very long time, and using that kind of inner learning to get a better understanding of how they lived their lives would be wonderful. Maybe I could even learn some of the ancient healing arts, to help myself and others. Whoops— there I was, working again. But I felt better thinking about something that seemed useful. I didn't feel comfortable doing nothing but vacationing. My need to learn, to be productive, was much stronger than my desire to play.

⚬⚬⚬

That evening, our landlady told us of a local restaurant we would enjoy. After having spent the day exploring the ruins of ancient Greek culture, we felt eating at a place full of tourists wouldn't seem appropriate. In fact, we decided to go native.

What I liked right away about the restaurant was that it was well-lighted. No dark corners or mystery dinners here. While waiting for our food, we noticed that the tables were set up in a unique way. Men, old and young, sat on one side of what appeared to be a small dance floor. Women were on the other side. As dinner progressed, I noticed the men at one table looking over at us, constantly making eye contact with Kellee and me, smiling in a friendly way. We naturally smiled back. Later I realized this was their standard way of finding a date for the remainder of the evening.

After dinner, the most wonderful thing happened. The men who had been flirting with us got up and began to dance. Watching them jump up and down, swaying from side to side, we realized we were witnessing a form of mating dance. The younger men would flex their muscles, leap into the air, and come down on one foot, only to jump up again. Truly it was a most sensual, sexy ritual as the dancers went faster and faster. I held my breath, totally caught up in the drama.

To my utter amazement, one of the men came over and grabbed my hand, bringing me into their dance circle. I did my best to keep up with them, but it was very strenuous. After only a few minutes, I struggled back to my chair, collapsing, gasping for breath. It was turning out to be the best night we had experienced so far. We were mixing it up with the locals and I felt wonderfully alive and sexy, something I hadn't felt in a long time. I wanted more.

Romance is everywhere in Greece. People have a very different attitude. Love, they believe, just like good wine, is to be savored. I was tempted by the man's interest, but more than that, I was flattered. No guys had come on to me in a long time. Of course, as Kellee so nastily pointed out, my suitor probably thought I was a rich American woman looking for a one-night stand with a dashing foreigner. Or, she ventured, he might want to come back to the States as the husband of a rich American woman. She certainly did know how to burst a bubble. Still, I didn't care. His attentions felt too good.

Somewhere deep inside though, I knew Kellee was right. And her suspicion fit right into my image of myself as unattractive to men. My track record with men was pretty bad. My self-esteem in regard to men was not high. That was not an area of my inner nature I really wanted to examine right then. Feeling sorry for myself was easier. Who would want me anyway?

We could have stayed in Crete for the entire time—except that I got a premonition, a dream, an intuitive flash. I had seen a sign for a tour to another island, called Santorini. For some unknown reason, I felt our going there was necessary and that we should do so as quickly as arrangements could be made. Too many times I have ignored my intuition and been sorry for it later. I wouldn't let this strong feeling go unheeded.

We settled our bill and said grateful goodbyes to our hostess. Quickly, we hopped on a tiny airplane that skimmed over the tops of the waves from island to island. In about an hour, we landed on Santorini.

Our luggage was dumped beneath a rusty barrel that had a sign identifying it as the baggage claim area. This whole idea might have been a mistake. Although we were told that the island was very modern and that we would be thrilled by the archaeological digs (which might have uncovered the lost city of Atlantis), I was beginning to have my doubts. My first impression was giving me grief. What in the world was my intuition doing? How could this island have produced the psychic pull I felt? Why were we here?

There was no airport lounge. We just climbed out of the plane, retrieved our bags, and there we were, waiting for a taxi. One of the two taxis on the small island finally came chugging up to where we were standing. With a toothy grin, the driver hopped out, starting loading our bags, and cheerfully told us his name was George. He was very proud that he spoke good English. He asked if we were Americans. Remembering the warning from our first plane ride, we told him we were from Canada. He said no, he didn't believe us, that we were from California in the U.S.A. How did he know? I guess they were smarter than we gave them credit for. No one ever seemed to believe we were Canadians, anyway. Well, everyone appeared to like people from California, and they usually even expressed a desire to live there. We began to realize that everyone thought California was the land of milk and honey. Or at least the land of surfer dudes and blonde, bronzed, beautiful women. Not to mention, Hollywood. Everyone loved movies!

George took us under his wing. When he heard we were interested in seeing the dig site, he changed course immediately. Concerned, we told him we wanted to go to the hotel first, to freshen up.

"No time, lady," he replied. The site would be closing soon, and since we were going to be on the island for only a short time, less than twenty-four hours, it was now or never.

❦

Santorini is a small part of what remains of a great land mass that was blown up by a huge volcanic explosion somewhere around 1500 B.C., a blast many times more powerful than that of St. Helen's.

Most of the archeological site was under a tin roof, protecting those who were working the dig, but also preserving the structures. It was incredible, even more spectacular than the one we visited on Crete. So much of everything was still intact. I was amazed to see the intricate spout systems built right into the structures. They collected precious rain water, which flowed into large, beautifully decorated, pottery jugs. The people, with their communal kitchens and artistic creations on the walls, were obviously a complex and advanced culture. I was in awe. All my beliefs about people in the ancient past were falling by the wayside as we strolled through the avenues of this ancient, abandoned city. Could this have been Atlantis? The paintings on the walls certainly depicted a civilization in harmony with nature. Pictures of dolphins as well as scenes of dancing and playing were evident in every building.

While roaming through the ruins we could overhear one of the tour guides explaining the significance of the structures. At one point, a small marker covered with fresh roses was the focus of conversation. Here, the man who discovered the archaeological site had died. He was buried where he fell, to honor him and his find. Mentally I said a quick thank-you to his remains.

This was, I learned, one of the richest archeological finds in recent history. I wondered if the man who discovered it knew his contribution to science and the world would be remembered and respected. I hoped so. What an honor, I thought. Where, I asked myself, would I be buried? An interesting question.

Our faithful, happy driver was waiting for us when we emerged from the tin-roofed building. He was happy we enjoyed the site. He obviously was proud of it.

"I must make a stop and pick up some people," he said to us as he began to drive away. I was suspicious. This didn't sound right. For some reason, we weren't in control of our driver. It was as if we got in a cab at Kennedy Airport, said we wanted to go to the United Nations Building, and were told we were going to Atlantic City, instead.

"What people?" I asked, trying to be somewhat authoritative, but he went on anyway.

His "people" turned out to be the daughter of the deceased archaeologist. She was a renowned archaeologist in her own right and a lovely woman. I was very self-conscious. Here, in the flesh, was the daughter of a fallen hero. She spoke English like a native of the British Isles. Her name was Annie.

We soon discovered she taught at the American University in Athens. She was here, for just the day, with a woman from Sweden who was filming a documentary for Swedish television about her and her father's work. Both of them squeezed in beside Kellee. The honor of sitting in the front seat was bestowed on me. George had taken a liking to me, although I was unaware of it at the time.

On the way to the hotel, Annie and I began discussing the cultural mythology of the Atlantians. I mentioned my understanding that they had used gemstones and crystals for healing. Annie became very animated. I could tell she was intrigued that I knew about the healing arts of the ancient culture. While we were talking, our eyes kept meeting and, as if some kind of telepathy were taking place, I was given reinforcement of my knowledge about healers who lived so long ago.

She and I hit it off immediately, like kindred spirits. She invited us to come to Athens to visit her, where she would show me some of her findings. I was overjoyed to find someone who knew so much about the secrets of the healing arts in ancient times, for the idea of advancing my knowledge to help others was intoxicating. I began to understand why I had such a strong pull to come to Santorini. It may have been just to meet this woman. Certainly it was a magical meeting. She had not been to Santorini for years and, like us, was only here for this one day. It must have been destiny that we met.

The feeling of being in a play, scripted long before I was aware, was overpowering. It was as if time were standing still. I knew instinctively that my being there on that day was part of the path my life was following. Whatever else was to happen, the trip had been worth it. Meeting Annie was a highlight, as well as a confirmation of my own inner ability to be aware of the universe around me.

The name of our hotel was the Atlantis. Naturally. Why was I not surprised? Although the tourist season had not yet arrived in the Greek Isles, our not having planned ahead was still risky. We hadn't made reservations and, in fact, didn't know if we'd be able to find a place to stay at all—unless we realized this trip was made possible by Something that knew more about what was going on than we did. Reservations aren't necessary on the road to enlightenment.

The nearby village was on a cliff about three hundred feet about the water. I noticed only a few cars, since most people walked. A great many donkeys were in service, however, carrying various bundles for their owners.

The lifestyle was idyllic, or at least what we had seen was. The cliffs overlooked a remarkably brilliant blue bay, so clear I felt as though I could see all the way to the bottom. Resting almost in the middle of the bay, however, was a truly frightening sight. A deadly cone, hundreds of yards wide, evidence of the volcano, lay there—nearly flat, pitch black, and totally barren of all life. The only activity was a thin column of smoke or steam, escaping from the gaping hole in the center, a constant reminder of the potential destructive power lurking below the serenely blue water. This was not a dead volcano, but a sleeping giant, waiting to be awakened from its centuries of silence, ready to complete the job it started those thousands of years ago. Looking at it gave me chills. So quiet, so peaceful—yet the danger was real, cleverly hidden under the sea.

The presence of the volcano gave an energy to the surrounding land and its people that was unmistakable, almost as if humanity was saying to nature, "I know you're dangerous, but I just don't care. I'm going to live my life." Their situation is not unlike that of people living along the San Andreas Fault in California. Someday California, or some parts of it along that geologic fault, will be jolted by an enormous earthquake and large portions of the area may end up flooded by water from the inrushing Pacific Ocean. At least, that's what various experts suggest.

The day stretched out languidly and peacefully. I was in an altered state of awareness, one in which time seemed sometimes changed, molded, slowed, and even stopped. These were precious moments. Time was doing us a great favor by not going so fast. Kellee and I found a wonderful balcony overlooking the bay and the sleeping, fire-breathing volcano dragon. Bright, colorful flowers bordered our corner. We sat, squarely facing the volcano, laughing and relaxing as we sipped some of the local wine. A feeling of belonging settled in my soul. I breathed deeply and was content. Even with extreme potential danger a stone's throw away, I was at peace.

As a reward for George's kindness, we invited him to his favorite restaurant for dinner. That he had taken a liking to me was now obvious, and though I was flattered, I wasn't that interested. But his friendship was welcome.

The sun was about to slip over the edge, heading toward the other side of the world, so Kellee and I decided to get ready for dinner. She won the coin toss and got the first shower. I decided to step out on the little two-person balcony. The sky was mauve, pink, grey, and blue, swimming with magical colors—the shades and hues reflected off the darkening blue-black bay. Yet I could still make out the outline of the volcano, its steam now more evident against the darkening backdrop. The wind was drifting in, like a gentle lover, stroking the side of my face.

Suddenly and without warning, the world and the room seemed to explode. My first thought was that the volcano had erupted. Then I realized that the Greek church, which was touching the outside of our hotel's side wall, had come to life. A series of bells, maybe as many as ten or twelve, were going off to say farewell to the sun, which just started to disappear into the sea.

Kellee, who had been shampooing her hair in the shower, came running out into the room. Her face had the look of a startled deer. The vibration from the bells had shaken her so greatly in the shower that she thought we were having an earthquake! Seeing shampoo streaming down her face onto the floor in a frothy puddle made me start to laugh. As soon as she realized she wasn't in immediate danger, and how silly she must look, she too began to laugh. We continued until our sides ached. The bells finally stopped and Kellee finished her shower.

I returned to the doorway of the balcony, with the colors of the sky even more intense, yet darker with the fading light. The beauty of it was magnified when I heard the Greek priest begin to sing. His voice, sweet, pure, and strong, came drifting back on the waves of the balmy breeze. At that moment, I thought this must be what heaven is like. Tears of joy and unbelievable contentedness washed over me. What a way to end our only day on Santorini.

Some say it is an enchanted island. They won't get an argument from me. The day was truly enchanted. I felt as though I was in exactly the right place at exactly the right time. I was in tune with nature, and it felt wonderful. My only regret was that I couldn't stay like this.

George arrived just when he had promised. He was dressed in black slacks and a clean, starched white shirt. We also dressed up for the occasion. We felt festive and were looking forward to a celebration of life and new friendship.

We asked George to take us to his favorite place to eat. We drove down to the other side of the island, where the sand on the beach is jet black. Little fishing boats, painted red, green, blue, and white, had been pulled onto the beach for the night. The moon was beginning to make its presence known, its light sufficient for us to see the florescent white wave tops hitting the black sand, gently and rhythmically. It was a wondrous sight, on a day I thought couldn't get any better.

The restaurant faced the beach. As we walked up a few steps and into the main dining area, George called out to announce our entrance. Within seconds, a huge man and an equally large woman came up to greet us. When George introduced Kellee and me, they grabbed and kissed us on both cheeks. We were now family. They didn't speak any English, but George was doing a great job of translating. Before being seated, we were taken on a tour of the kitchen and introduced to the cook.

The cook, delighted at our interest, started dipping his fingers into the different pots and bowls he was preparing. Without hesitation or any formality, he placed the food, and his fingers, into our startled o-shaped mouths. We were getting a real treat…to be able to try out the food before ordering. They certainly wanted our dinner to be the best they had to offer.

The food and the people were all wonderful. Sitting at the table, I felt as though we were at the home of dear friends, sharing good food and laughter. Kellee and I looked at each other and just smiled. When in Rome, eh? Only this was better. The warmth and love these people offered us was genuine, and no amount of money or social status on earth could have brought forth the response we were privileged to receive.

The owners joined us for dinner, sharing their best wines as well. The evening was getting off to a wonderful start. Again, the feeling of having been pulled to this tiny island in a strange sea settled on my shoulder.

After a while, we noticed some people coming up the steps. As the owners excused themselves, George, Kellee, and I returned to our food and drink. Within a few seconds, however, Kellee nudged me with her elbow. "Look at that," she whispered, nodding toward the door.

Approximately fifteen blind people were coming in for dinner. Some with canes and other with sighted guides. We couldn't believe it. Could that many visually impaired people possibly live on this tiny island? Our curiosity increased to an unbearable degree. Then, to top it all, we heard them speaking English. Not American English, but British English.

That's it. We had to investigate. I made Kellee go over first. When she came back she said they were all from England, and this was their first trip outside that county as a group. They came to explore the archaeological digs. We were astonished and amazed. Now I knew why we had to come to this island on this particular day.

They had been asking around for the best restaurant and this was the one they selected. Out of all the places in the world, they picked this one. It occurred to me that I could not get lost on my path. Not with this much cooperation from the Universe. The work I was doing was right and this seemed to prove it.

We joined their party and had one hell of a good time, talking, comparing vision problems, laughing, and just relishing the evening. It was magical, and it reinforced my desire to help myself and those with vision problems to live life to the fullest. With or without sight! These people were certainly doing exactly that. I had to remind myself that I, too, had a vision problem, yet here we all were, living life.

The next day, less than twenty-four hours after our arrival, we left our little treasure island.

It may have been a short visit, but it was one of the most significant experiences I ever had while traveling. Time did expand for us that day and night. Someday, I want to return to Santorini and stay longer. It is one of the few places on earth I physically yearn for and miss.

Back to England. Cold, grey, windy. We were thrilled with our tanned bodies. We looked so healthy that we didn't mind the bleak English spring. Our class was large and it kept us busy from early morning to late night. The people were fabulous. I'd heard the British were reserved, but didn't find it to be true at all. Their wonderful sense of humor and willingness to share their inner feelings completely destroyed the myth of their being aloof. Maybe it was our common bond or maybe it was the way our experience together unfolded. Regardless, our class was one of the most enlightening and powerful I ever conducted. Twenty people of different backgrounds and races made it a very eclectic group as well.

The oldest gentleman, Amrit, was a revered Hindu priest who happened to be a world-renowned Sanskrit scholar. His dear friend and disciple brought him to the class every day before going to work. Amrit was a fountain for information and wouldn't hesitate to stand up at various times to explain the origins of certain words. (For instance, he explained one day that "God" and "Eye" in ancient Sanskrit had the same root meaning. We didn't entirely understand the importance of his telling us that, but the matter was important to him.)

Amrit had glaucoma, a condition that can lead to total blindness, and in his case, apparently had. Due to his advanced age, conventional medicine wasn't helpful.

But something about Amrit made me think, "Hmmm, what's wrong with this picture?" At first, I couldn't put my finger on it, then about three days into the program, the answer came to me like a florescent tube flashing on. He always kept his eyes closed! No matter if he was talking, walking, eating, or just sitting at rest, his eyes were shut.

When the time came for me to work privately with Amrit, I asked him about his closed eyes. I learned that years before, around the time of the onset of the glaucoma, he started keeping them closed due to his discomfort from lights in general and glare in particular. Keeping them closed had become habitual. In fact, he was not now even aware they were closed. He no longer tried to see at all, and went about his daily business with his eyes closed tight. People naturally assumed he was totally blind, as he himself did.

Having realized what was happening, I asked Amrit to open his eyes—and he reported seeing traces of movement. He was not totally blind! After several days of my continuing gentle reminders, he began to keep his eyes open consistently and was able to see! It was not clear vision, nor very practical, but it was helpful in some situations. To those with impaired visual function, a little is a great deal—certainly better than total blindness, even if it's only the ability to distinguish daylight from darkness. His joy and the look on his disciple's face lifted my spirits considerably—especially when his disciple reported that Amrit, after the third day, was able to eat his meal by sight, rather than by his usual touch-and-feel method!

Amrit still had glaucoma but as a result of the training program, the discomfort he felt from glare was greatly reduced, as was his need to keep his eyes closed.

It was no miracle cure, though both Amrit and his friend the disciple wanted to credit me with one. It was just a matter of observation. I believed anyone could have recognized the problem. Then again, when a person assumed someone is blind, why bother telling him his eyes are closed? I just happened to be the one who questioned the totality of his blindness.

Our class even produced a love story. Ben and Julia, both lovely, lonely, and sight-impaired, had no difficulty finding each other. This class was making me wish I were a participant instead of the teacher. The students seemed to be having all the fun. I began to feel a little left out.

Another of the students was a successful rock music producer. He was the most kind and sensitive of all the people I had known in that line of work. By his own admission, though, he had not been so nice until he took the class. It led him to change his attitude and even his lifestyle, away from self-destruction and self-pity. To witness the healing of his soul during the two weeks we were together was an experience that will stay with me the rest of my life.

His ability to articulate what he was feeling emotionally gave us all deep insight into ourselves. Not only did he begin to heal his own spirit, but he also contributed greatly to the healing and strengthening of the spirit of each person in attendance. To my great sorrow, he did not get much, if any, improvement in his visual function. That didn't seem to dampen his spirit, however.

A year later, he shared with me that he received a greater gift than sight. He found peace within himself and his world. He told me he felt his spirit had been healed. That seemed much more important than sight, at least to him. I understood what he meant, for that is the goal I, myself, have been striving for all these many years. My student had truly surpassed his teacher. Now I could learn from him. What he gained, I wanted to have as well.

⟨❧⟩

The two weeks passed much too quickly. We all became very close, and—as usual—the only sensible thing to do was to have a party celebrating the end of our time together. Two blocks away was a great Greek restaurant. It seemed fitting to Kellee and me that we conclude our first English course with a Greek dinner party—especially because of our recent experience on Santorini.

Having twenty sight-impaired people move en masse to the restaurant required that friends and family members be invited as well. Instead of twenty-two, there were at least forty. The restaurant closed its doors in the early afternoon to accommodate us all. The tables were arranged in a U-formation, and we all fit nicely. Our agreement called for paying the checks separately, so we each ordered exactly what we wanted, including, as it turned out, enough bottles of wine to make it a festive occasion.

After the main course, with its conversations and laughter, the time came to be serious. I had decided to buy rosebuds, one for each of our graduates. As I went from individual to individual, praising their courage and their success, I presented each with a single rose. The rosebud symbolized hope, I explained. At first, the bud is tiny, like one's limited sight. As time passes, the rosebud blossoms, as does one's vision, both inner and outer.

It was a very emotional afternoon, and we all shared much love and gratitude.

I believed the party was over, but I was in for another surprise. Every one of our participants stood, each in turn saying thanks, and telling us something special. Kleenex was used in abundance, I can assure you. The music producer, a successful, usually hard-nosed businessman, was the last to share his feelings. His speech was eloquent and touching. He praised the courage of the group and swore he would never feel sorry for himself again. He had only to draw on his memory of these past two weeks to give himself an edge in beating depression and self-pity. He wept openly and unashamedly. We all joined him for a magnificent collective hug.

After such an emotion afternoon, I needed to do something special for myself. Kellee was on her way back to the States for a class reunion. I had a long trip ahead, to Sweden and Germany. With a three-day weekend coming up, I decided to take the night train to Scotland. Hattie, one of my students, who was once married to an Italian diplomat, had friends in a little village above Glasgow, on the west coast of Scotland. With a simple phone call, I set up my travel and lodging plans. Hastily packing and hurrying to Victoria Station, I just made the last night train heading north.

16

EVERY CLOUD HAS A RADIOACTIVE LINING

Teaching a class, particularly one so wonderful and emotionally moving as the one I had just completed, required that I follow it up with time off. Years earlier, I learned to anticipate a let-down when I had been so high. After having shared deeply with the class and been part of their success, if I didn't plan something special for myself, depression would come to visit for at least two or three days.

Every class had its own personality, but all had one thing in common. We became very close in a short time. If we dealt with every aspect of the program, little time remained for small talk. We dug deep down and covered a great deal of personal territory. When the two weeks were over and the time came for everyone to go home, we all felt as though we were losing close friends. I needed to distance myself from that intensity and give myself a reward after each course was finished. Sometimes a short trip to the beach or a small dinner party with friends or family would do the trick. But this time, after this kind of high-level experience, I needed much more. These people got under my skin. We had bridged many differences and achieved not only physical improvement but also spiritual healings of the soul as an added bonus.

A train trip to Scotland was the perfect answer, and it gave me a three-day weekend for a vacation.

The sleeper car was a waste of time, not to mention money. The sleeping compartment itself was so tiny that I had to stuff my luggage between the wall and the little shelf of a bed. Like a total idiot, I changed into my nightgown, which was a big mistake, since the beds—narrow as a park bench and just as comfortable—were oriented at right angles to the length of the car and, therefore, the direction of the train. Every time the train took off, I rolled halfway out of the bed. When the train came to a stop, I rolled back toward the wall. Stop and go, stop and go. The only time I slept was when the train stopped over for two hours in one of the stations. I should have saved the fare. I would have been better off fully dressed, sitting out in the club car, instead of pretending I could fall asleep on that humpty-dumpty train. But what did I know?

By morning, I had changed back into street clothes and was anxious to get a peek at Scotland. The mystery and mystique of the place caught my fancy in advance, and I wanted to get a glimpse of the legendary landscape.

At the first opportunity, I stuck my head out the window. Mother Nature didn't disappoint me one bit. The train was traveling at high speed and my looking out that window was like putting my head in an Arctic wind tunnel. But it gave me a perfect view of the surrounding countryside.

That view was spectacular. Hardly a house, car, or human in sight, as far as the eye could see. Ancient mountains, worn smooth from the ages, were magnificent. Topped with a whipped-cream-like snow (accounting for the Arctic temperature), they were abundant on our route. I didn't know if it was weather, but the vegetation looked dense and matted, almost surrealistic—like an old painting that had lost its first blush of color.

Happy as a dog sniffing the air during a ride in its master's car, I was transfixed. I felt as if I had come home. To have that kind of feeling surprised me, as my heritage is Irish, not Scottish.

My destination was Durror of Apin, a small, sleepy village of about three hundred, with its structure nestled around a beautiful Lok. Lok means lake, and this particular one, according to information I picked up locally, was fed by the Bermuda current from the South Atlantic.

I was met at the train station by the staff of the inn where I would be staying. My hostess was the niece of the owner, and she cleared up my confusion about feeling I had come home. She told me a great many Irish settlers, in times long ago, had migrated from here in Scotland. Ah, that explained it. Some long-forgotten contributor to my unique gene pool must have been Scottish.

The bed-and-breakfast inn looked like an old castle, but of a simpler kind than the monstrous Gothic types I'd seen in most travel brochures of Europe. This one was livable. My room, huge by any standards, had a giant feather bed that enabled me to sink in, deep and toasty warm, giving me the feeling I was being held by someone who loved me. It's difficult to find a good substitute for a warm body lying next to you in bed, and this was as close as I had yet come. My first thought after plopping myself in the middle of the welcoming bed was to spend my three-day vacation snuggling up to the mattress. After my experience of sleeplessness on the train, I was exhausted. My hostess said she would let me sleep for two hours and wake me for breakfast. That suited me fine.

The weight of the world was getting lighter with each passing hour. The sense of congestion that came from feeling millions of energy fields, the inhabitants of a busy, bustling metropolis like London, was slipping off my spirit like a satin shirt. This was what I called "Stress Reduction." I had never taken a vacation by myself. This was just a short one, but I was savoring every second.

After a wonderful Scottish breakfast, I ventured outside and decided to look around. The mist was beginning to lift, though the morning was still cool. The inn was off a main roadway which was not used often. Rolling hills, I saw, encircled the Lok. I decided to explore them, taking a well-worn path that led off the paved road. I pulled my sweater and coat tighter and started off and upward.

It was April. Spring comes late in Scotland. The creek flowing by the path—a strong runoff from the melting snow hidden higher up—was rushing noisily, producing an icy mist above it. The banks were steep and slippery, with many shades of green vegetation. The path was wide enough for me to follow without difficulty. Winding its way toward the top, it suddenly veered across a small, smooth stone bridge constructed long ago.

Not from being tired, but as if guided to do so, I stopped in the middle of the bridge. Turning to view the magnificent scenery below, I leaned against the ancient rocks that made a three-foot-high guardrail. The sun was behind me, over the top of the hill I was climbing. Sheep, mostly silent, grazed head-down, busy at their job of survival. Trees, a few with leaves, dotted the landscape here and there. The grass that coated the hill was rich and dark green, almost emerald. Appreciating its beauty, I was immensely grateful for having been able to keep my sight as long as I had.

After a few minutes of silent meditation and gratitude, I turned to look up toward my goal. What I saw made all my previous visual experiences insignificant. A small but well defined bare tree was lit up—astonishingly. Thousands of star-like lights dotted the thin, bare branches, as though they were sparkling diamonds. The vision took my breath away. I realized that countless dewdrops had caught the illumination of the sun for a few brief moments, and it was a most magical sight, as if this tree was sparkling just for me. Standing transfixed, I took in the view, thinking that somehow God was talking to me. Soon, the bright pin-lights started to fade. For those few seconds, this tiny tree wore so much brilliant jewelry that the queens of history would have been jealous.

These magical interludes were putting my spirit in such a state that I thought I would burst with happiness. I hadn't been in Scotland for more than three hours and already the land shared its treasures. If indeed there are fairies and little people with magical powers, they had been putting on a fabulous show for me. Tears of pure joy slid down my cheeks.

Not wanting to break the spell, I remained still. Then, from far down the hillside, a loud and sorrowful wail brought me out of my reverie. At first it sounded like a child crying. For some strange reason, that cry triggered something deep inside me. I felt an urgency to locate its source.

As I hurried toward what sounded for all the world like a plea for help, I slipped once on the wet path, then struggled to my feet. When I neared the source of crying, I realized it was not a human, but a little lamb.

Now, I'm not the farm-girl type, and my personal experience with lambs has been mostly at a dinner table. So I really didn't know what, if anything, to do. But the cry for help was unmistakable, even in animal language. The closer I got, the more I realized that this little baby had lost its way. A part of me felt as if I had been crying similarly. Not recently, but a long time ago. The feeling quickly passed.

Finally, I was able to see the lamb's predicament, as it was stuck on the edge of the steep riverbank, with many bushes blocking its access to safety. It seemed ready to fall into the freezing water below. Without hesitation, I plowed my way down, holding onto branches and bushes I hoped were anchored well into the earth. Reaching out, I grabbed the lamb by one of its front legs and began to pull it up the steep slope. Struggling and confused, the little creature resisted. Finally, in response to my gentle but urgent coaxing, he began to cooperate in my rescue effort. After a few minutes, the two of us were back on solid ground. With a little nudge of his nose—I think he was saying thanks—he was off and running. He never looked back.

I watched until he was out of sight. I felt good. The planet had given me many gifts that day. Memories of a wonderful Scottish morning stay with me yet. Things seemed so simple there on the cool hillside, far from home.

⚬⚬⚬

Coming back to the B & B was rewarding. A huge, roaring fire in the living room greeted me. A lovely wingback chair was at the right distance from the flames. Perfect to give warmth and comfort. A brandy snifter held a few fingers of golden brown drink that smelled like Scotch and felt like liquid fire traveling into my tummy. That's the way to warm up in Scotland. A person's bones get cold in that climate.

The three-day vacation was over too soon. The time came to move on, since Reba had established speaking engagements all over Sweden for me. With a sad farewell and a determination to return someday to Scotland, I headed for Glasgow, where I was to catch a plane to Stockholm.

Greece had been my training ground for sticking my head in the sand. I hadn't watched television for nearly a week, but I had a set in my room at the inn. While packing to leave, I decided to turn it on. The BBC usually has good coverage of what's happening in the world, and I thought I should catch up on things.

Libya—less than 150 miles from the Greek island where I stayed—had been bombed by President Reagan. Now I realized that with the way things were in the world, anything could have happened while I was happily herding lost sheep in the wilderness.

Could there be more? I waited.

❦

The BBC announcer was almost excited for a change. The interviews shifted back and forth and I realized something terrible had happened. An electronic blink and there was a familiar American newscaster, nearly hysterical, telling of thousands killed by an out-of-control nuclear power plant in the Soviet Union.

My mouth felt like cotton as I sat down with a thud on the bed in front of the TV. Clothes were ready to be packed; I dropped them on the floor. For the moment, I forgot everything.

The American seemed close to losing control, while the BBC announcer was calm, composed, and sitting very still as he kept the audience up to date on the biggest nuclear accident the world had yet to experience. The difference between the BBC announcer and the American announcer was almost funny, and maybe it actually would have been if the situation weren't so deadly.

Chernobyl, I learned, had succeeded in doing what, a few years earlier, we were afraid would happen at Three Mile Island in Pennsylvania. Chernobyl had gone ballistic, spewing its deadly, invisible radiation into the skies over the western parts of the Soviet Union. Memories of the movie The China Syndrome flashed in my mind.

The newscasts were sketchy and dependent on the Swedish government for most of their information. I was confused because I wasn't exactly sure where Sweden was. But the country I was supposed to fly to on this very day was somehow involved in this horrid accident. As the news unfolded, I understood that it was the Swedes who blew the whistle on the Soviets, as Swedish airspace and land were showing increased amounts of radiation. They—not the Soviet Union—were the first to tell the world what happened.

Should I fly to Stockholm? I knew little about radiation, except that it was bad. I was at war with the part of me that wanted to fly to Sweden and fulfill my commitment to Reba, and the part of me that wanted to run away to safety and not go near the danger zone. My schedule had been established months in advance. People were depending upon me to show up. On the other hand, I was scared to death. Was I going to fry in Sweden? Would I meet my commitments only to die a slow, painful death due to radiation exposure? It was a hard decision. The newscasters weren't much help.

I really had no choice. I had to go. The tickets had been purchased, and if there was a danger, I was certain the airlines and the countries involved wouldn't let people travel. At least, that's how I conned myself into climbing on the plane. Little did

I realize that I would be suffering the consequences for many years to come.

17

THE INQUISITION

It was a smooth flight, with an overnight stop in Copenhagen. Arrival was scheduled for the next afternoon in Sweden. I put the fear of radiation behind me, praying that the people around the nuclear disaster site would be spared. The news was grim and without knowing how serious this accident was, I could only hope for the best.

The hotel was old and elegant. My room looked out over the main public square of the city. This was Copenhagen's heart. It was beautiful, surrounded by very old buildings. Looking down, I saw a group of people in white maintenance uniforms; they were working, apparently scrubbing and washing the cobblestone street and mosaic terraces. From my distance and with my eyesight, I thought it odd. Then I remembered that pigeons leave droppings in these types of city squares. I had heard that this often presented health problems to passersby. How wonderful of the Danes, I thought. They were out there scrubbing off the pigeon leavings. A nasty job, but thank goodness someone was doing it. They even appeared to be wearing breathing masks. Hah, I said to myself. Pigeon doo-doo appears to be more dangerous than that nasty old radiation from Russia. Turning away, I felt somehow safer. You can see pigeon droppings. You can't avoid radiation, even with the best of sight.

With a light heart, I decided to go exploring. Then, on the street, as I approached the workers in white, I saw more clearly what was on their uniforms. Oh my God! They weren't washing down bird droppings, they were cleaning away the silent poison from the sky, Chernobyl's doo-doo. The symbol they wore was the clear, unmistakable international warning: CAUTION, NUCLEAR RADIATION.

My mind reeled as I ran back to the safety of my hotel room. Now I was really frightened. However, people didn't seem to be in a panic. Still, there were those workers. What could it all mean? I hated being alone and thousands of miles away from my family and friends right then. I didn't want to be an adult. Grown-ups were clearly screwing up the world, and I didn't seem to be able to do a damned thing about it. Except to be about my business. The next morning, I was on the flight to Stockholm.

⊙✖∋

The invisible poison knew nothing of borders. The northernmost area of Sweden, for example, is part of the geographic region called Lapland, located well within the Arctic Circle. Lapland is the home of the reindeer. Or used to be. Hundreds of herds had to be put to death as a result of the fallout from Chernobyl. The reindeer not only pull Santa's sleigh, but they are also a major source of food for the people in Scandinavia. It would be a lean winter for many. The Russians weren't the only ones to suffer losses.

❦

Seeing Reba and her family was wonderful. Being with a family made me miss Ru all the more, as this was the longest we had ever been apart. I missed the big guy—tall, skinny, and gangly, the light of my life. The only thing that eased my aching and lonely heart was when I was able to talk about him, which I did as often as I could work it into conversation or a speech. He was my anchor as well as my rudder.

From what I observed, Sweden is one of the world's most thoughtful countries where the welfare of its citizens is concerned. Especially for those who are less fortunate. Every street corner had clicking signal lights to let the blind and visually impaired know when crossing the street was safe. Elevators announced the floor number and had raised numerals on the buttons. I cannot begin to count how many times I have ridden up and down in an elevator waiting for someone to get on to tell me if I pushed the right button and when the desired stop arrived. Talk about your yo-yo. I probably could get into the Guinness Book of World Records for miles uselessly traveled on elevators. Not so in Sweden. Officials in the government seemed really to care about the difficulties faced by people with disabilities. They identified the problems, then found solutions that left those individuals able to retain their dignity.

Amazing. Simply amazing. It was one of the most refreshing, enlightening experiences in all my travels. If the language weren't so difficult and if the sun shone more in the fall and winter, I would consider moving to Sweden permanently. But those are lots of ifs. Maybe someday our government will study the way Sweden works with its physically challenged citizens. I saw no homeless on the streets of Sweden, either.

The speaking engagement came and went; my ideas and work were wellreceived. Although there was some minor controversy, all in all things went well. I would apparently be invited back to teach a course later in the year.

Now, I was ready to travel again. I suppose I was really ready to go home, as I was tired of living out of suitcases, but home was not coming along for me yet.

⚜

Germany was a surprise. Reba decided to travel with me, since she made the invitation possible in the first place. Her position in the Green Party government gave her some credibility with the organizers of the annual International RP Convention. I'm sure that is why I was invited. Plus, Reba's daughter did so well in getting around by herself after completing the program that Reba was able to pursue her own dream of getting into politics. Her enthusiasm was certainly transmitted to the leader of the conference.

The gathering was being held in Bad Nauheim, a little resort village about an hour out of Frankfurt. The facility was huge and attendance was expected to be in the neighborhood of seven hundredplus. Scientists, doctors, and people with RP from all over the world were joining together for three days. At least half of those in attendance were either afflicted with RP or were friends and family members of people who were afflicted.

Registration was a madhouse. Check-in guides, fluent in three or more languages, were stationed about the room. The many blind or visually impaired people wandering around made this a unique, noisy, and confusing registration process. The conference hadn't even begun, and I could tell that the people hosting the event were already stressed in a major way. I had to laugh a little and thought what a wonderful opportunity this would be to break into a demonstration of

Stress Management. Oh well, deep breathing for myself was about as much as I could handle at the time.

I was excited and nervous—and could never have prepared for the welcome I received. When Reba and I identified ourselves, I noticed that one of the table attendants signaled to someone behind us. Not thinking this would involve me, I focused my attention on our room assignments and directions. But I should have been paying more attention.

The signal alerted the convention organizer, a German gentleman, of my arrival. In a few moments, he was at my side, out of breath, beet red in the face, looking as if he was ready to explode. He was trying to say something to me in English, but whatever it was, it was unintelligible to me. I had just become accustomed to people speaking English with a Swedish accent, and hadn't yet adjusted my ears to the very different sounds now coming at me. Sometimes my ears ached from trying so hard to hear and understand. Talk about eye strain. Has anyone ever thought about ear strain? I know I hadn't, not until I was traveling overseas.

The man was finally beginning to come into focus in the hearing portion of my brain. But it didn't make sense. Reba listened to him for a few minutes as well, and before I clearly understood what was happening, she went into a controlled but very powerful rage. Speaking in German, Swedish, and English, she was almost yelling at the poor fellow.

Apparently, he had been trying to reach me, but I was on the road traveling these last five weeks. Some of the "scientists," it seems, and especially the British and American doctors attending, requested that I not be allowed to speak to the assembly. They felt I wasn't a credible representative of the scientific community and would somehow taint the meeting.

What? I couldn't believe it.

Instead of getting wild and crazy like Reba, however, I became very calm. But my mind was spinning. What possible threat could I be to these people? I never made false claims about my program. All I ever said was fight. Fight the disease process with every ounce of strength. Fight the depression that comes with the invading darkness. Why would they object to this? None of the objectors ever talked to me directly, so how could they possibly make any determinations? What in the world were they afraid of?

The Conference people hadn't paid my way, nor were they covering the cost of the room. I traveled ten thousand miles, on my own money. The least they could do was to let me speak. That was Reba's argument and I had to agree.

The befuddled and stressed-out Conference leader finally came up with a plan. A lunchtime meeting would be held to determine if I had something that people wanted to hear. Later on, with me out of the room, a vote would be taken to decide whether I could participate. In other words, a mini-trial—or, more accurately, "inquisition"— was to be held. At least, that's how I felt about it. There would be a "special meeting," with ten of the scientific-medical people and ten from the RP side, none of whom had scientific or medical credentials. The moderator, a German woman who was to head the panel on which I was scheduled to speak, would be the tie-breaker, if that was necessary.

The meeting room had a long table, set for the twenty-two of us. The scientists took one side, the RP sufferers the other, leaving the moderator and me at either end. My heart was in my throat. When the waiter placed my plate in front of me, I thought I would lose my cool completely. They had chosen to serve blood-rare roast beef, some kind of potato, and peas. The bleeding meat made me want to gag. In some ways, I felt the beef lying on my plate represented my soul, now on display for a not-so-friendly crowd.

It reminded me of the saying that for every new idea, there are thousands of people vying to hold onto the old ones. Now I was beginning to know how Galileo felt. The medical view was a litany that there wasn't a cure, therefore no treatment for RP could even be discussed. I was a thorn in their side. They couldn't wait to pull me out. Funny, but I didn't resent them so much that day. In fact, I began to feel a little sorry for them. Trying to put myself in their shoes, I imagined how some doctors must feel when they diagnose a patient with an incurable or untreatable disease. It has to hurt. Maybe that's why they tend to harden themselves with a shield of indifference and predictable, abrupt dismissal. Then they don't have to get personally involved and they save themselves the pain and anguish the patients and their families face. Not all are like that, but many have hardened their hearts.

All of a sudden I didn't hate them anymore. That's when it began to dawn on me why I was such a threat. If I was right—that something can be done—then they would have to rethink their entire position, including their belief system. And that is one of the most difficult things to rethink—a well-established belief system.

The session went on for nearly an hour. The attack from the medical-scientific group lost its intensity toward the end of the meeting. My initial anger and fear disappeared after my internal understanding of their thought process. After covering the bloody plate with my napkin, I came to peace within myself.

Most of the scientific types were trying hard to make me contradict myself or say something stupid or wrong. But it just wasn't working for them. The others, those with RP, had more intimate and searching questions for me. Since I had RP myself, no one could deny my personal experience. In the past, as a way to discredit my views, some doctors even made statements that I didn't have anything wrong with my eyes. But they just had to look at my retinas and the answer was clear. I have always been willing to let them take a peek.

My own experience with my program is what I share. Never claiming a cure, I have nothing to hide, and although I cannot always answer scientific questions to their satisfaction, they cannot deny my personal experience of success.

Members of the medical-scientific community have certain viewpoints that are outdated and have been for over a quarter of a century. Yet, for many reasons, they still cling to those moldy ideas. Their belief system reminds me of the story of a great teacher who is outside on the sidewalk on his hands and knees looking for lost keys one afternoon. Several of his students come by. Witnessing his plight, they ask if they can help. The teacher accepts their offer. Soon, they are all searching for the teacher's keys. Finally, one of the students asks the Great Master exactly where he lost them.

"In the house," is his reply.

"Why then, Master, do you look out in the street?"

"The light is much better out here," is his logical response.

Modern (and I use that term loosely) medicine is still looking where the light is better. It is, in general, using the Western philosophic model laid down several hundred years ago by thinkers in

Europe who declared that the mind and the material world are two entirely separate entities. Their ideas were essentially satisfactory for the time and paved the way for civilization to make great progress. But the picture they painted wasn't the whole story.

For example, early in our own century, physicists using the rigorous methods of their own discipline in pursuit of ultimate knowledge of the material world, startled themselves by discovering that, in certain crucial ways, the mind and the material world appear not to be entirely separate. The only problem is that much of the official medical establishment remains rooted in the old ways and, in fact, tends to be hostile toward approaches which claim interrelatedness between the mind and the material world (which usually means "the mind and the body").

Until changes in our awareness take place, most of us will still look to the men and women of science for guidance and wisdom, especially (and appropriately) in the areas of health and disease. When something goes wrong, we'll go to a specialist. That's what we've been taught. That's what I do. But sometimes, especially when something affects my eyes, satisfactory answers don't exist. The time has come also to look elsewhere for those answers—like inside ourselves. The light's not as good, but that's where much of what we seek is to be discovered.

These thoughts were going through my mind and I was no longer intimidated by the collection of scientific antagonists in the room. After an hour of questions and answers, I was asked to leave the room for the vote.

The result was interesting. The vote was ten for and ten against. Want to guess which ones were against? Well, the woman moderator was the tie-breaker. Her vote was in my favor. The scientists and doctors were aghast and demanded a compromise. The situation was such that I would be seated on a panel with at least one Nobel Prize winner, with the chance that another would be there. If I were allowed to sit with these highly decorated and respected men, it might give me credibility I had not earned—or so reasoned my critics.

A compromise was reached that satisfied everyone. I had no say in the matter. I would be allowed to speak, but from the front of the platform, on the floor. I would not be allowed on stage with the Nobel Prize winners. Those conditions were fine with me, even though Reba thought it was an outrage. I was learning fast about the class order of the scientific community. As long as I had the opportunity to speak, however, I wouldn't mind if I had to swing from the chandelier.

But when the conference convened and the time finally came for my introduction, I wasn't so cool. My palms were sweating like little artesian wells and I could feel my face burning with extra blood flowing due to the increased pressure and additional adrenaline.

The meeting was being simultaneously translated into three languages: French, German, and English. That confused me at first and I required a little while to get accustomed to the format. I could hardly hear the translator's voice coming through the earpiece. Simultaneous translation, as I had learned on the previous occasions, certainly does speed up a meeting, though. On occasion, I turned the dial to hear what it all sounded like in other tongues. I was beginning to wish God hadn't done what he did in Babel. The world would be a much easier place to get along in if we all spoke the same language, I thought.

⸎

Finally, the moderator, the woman who cast the tiebreaking vote in the meeting, began to introduce me. In a surprising turn of events, she told the entire audience of the process we had gone through that led to my being allowed to speak. By so doing, she gave more credence to my speech, and more people probably paid attention. In having been separated from the panel and forced to speak from the floor, I was put in the position of being perceived as an underdog, a wronged person.

At that point in the conference, more people seemed to have been milling outside the lecture hall than sitting inside. But now I could hear them coming in from the lobby. The room was getting to the point of having standing room only. And it was my turn to speak. This was what I had been waiting to do for a long time.

To tell the truth, I don't remember what I said. The stress of the moment caused my memory to be unable to hold the exact details. But from the tremendous response I got, I must have reached those for whom I intended the presentation. Afterward, I was besieged by requests for information and literature. People wanted me to visit them in their own countries. I was pleased and amazed. It was beyond my wildest dreams.

Ongoing results of that one day's talk were fantastic. I was invited to develop programs in France, Germany, Spain, England, Sweden, and even Iceland, a country so remote I never imagined I might visit there. Trips to Canada and Brazil were also among the results of my work that day. The Convention was an amazing window of opportunity, and I went through it. It completely altered my life for the next five years, as I traveled and experienced peoples of cultures, religions, and races worldwide.

The privilege of getting to know these people has given me enduring hope and confidence to continue my efforts. From poor farmers in Brazil (who traveled thousands of miles to work with me) to a Supreme Court Justice in Sweden, their courage, their spirit, and their ability to change all impressed me tremendously. I am awed by their presence and I thank the stars each day that I have been blessed to meet and work with them all.

Even missing Ru during this trip was worth it. The empty space in my heart that never stopped missing my daughter was almost filled up by these wonderful people. My hope was always that I made a difference in their lives and contributed to them at least half of what they contributed back to me. Their courage is never far from my mind.

God has been generous to me, allowing me this gift of friendship with so many different people. Amazing, isn't it? Here I am, despite all the mistakes of my past, having done something really worthwhile. Not that I can take too much credit. After all, this path was established for me long before I started on my journey. I am particularly aware of that fact since my path includes a genetically transmitted eye disease that was passed down through at least five generations and was on its way to me many decades before I was born.

Every time I strayed off the path, my work would find me. As I see things, there is no denying that my destiny was preordained. Help was always near when I needed it most. Having had such poor eyesight most of my life, I always asked that any messages from the Great Beyond be in LARGE BOLD PRINT. My guides or angels or whoever they are have always complied, making my journey very clear most of the time. If I wasn't paying attention to the signs telling me where I should go and what I should be doing, the signs would trip me or fall on my heart to wake me up. Indeed, I think I have had a great deal f help along the way, and I am always thanking God for it.

18

STAR LIGHT, START BRIGHT

My visit to Germany for the RP Convention had been powerful, stressful, and rewarding. But it was not my first visit to that country. I first went there with my father when I was six months old. He was part of the Occupation Force in 1946 which helped Germany move beyond the era of World War II. I traveled there in the bowels of a transport ship, across the Atlantic, with my mother.

Now, I was returning yet again. My friend Dea organized a two-week class for me to teach in Freiburg, a bustling old city near the Black Forest mountains bordering Switzerland. Eight people wanted to attend. The oldest was a man who survived the war. His name was Adolf. The youngest were Patricia, who was twelve, and her brother Peter, a very active and endearing eight-year-old. Everybody in between made it a diversified group. Our goals, however, were the same…to improve sight, to prevent the further deterioration of sight.

Dea's friend Stephan, who was fully sighted, gave me his apartment and said I was welcome to live and work there. He moved most of his furniture into storage so we could use his living room for the course. I was amazed by his attitude, since he wasn't visually impaired. However, Dea was his dear friend. She did have RP and she told him how much my program had helped her. His generosity was without bounds and he contributed unselfishly to the success of our group.

Adolf didn't like me and made that clear from the beginning. I suspected his war-time prejudices and dislike of Americans still existed, and I was his target for the next two weeks. His attitude intimidated me at first, but I realized it was his problem, not mine. The other people wanted to succeed with the program, not engage in personal bickering. I finally stopped butting heads with Adolf and concentrated on the rest of the group. They were marvelous.

In my courses, I have worked with almost all the major ethnic and religious groups of the world. Being exposed to so many ways of life has been a wonderful experience, as people who come together for the single purpose of being able to see as well as possible seem to put aside petty prejudices and work with each other in a harmony rarely achieved in ordinary endeavors. As often happens, the members of our group bonded with each other in a matter of days. We quickly became a family, no matter what language was being spoken or how many different cultures or religions were represented.

Interestingly enough, Patricia, the twelve-year-old, bonded with Adolf, who found himself being a surrogate grandfather. They became inseparable as the days went by. His demeanor softened by the eighth day. He was smiling more and the obvious affection between the two of them was contagious.

We were all rooting for Patricia and Peter, the youngest two in the group, to benefit from the program. That was not uncommon—for the adults to want the children to do well. I felt it was a natural, instinctive act reflecting a desire to perpetuate the species. For example, the older members of the group didn't mind if I took Peter and Patricia first in the one-on-one therapies or if I gave them both a little extra attention. In fact, I was often encouraged by the group to do just that.

Most of the participants spoke English, but Dea and Stephan helped when translation was necessary. That made for slow going, though it got the job done. After using translators in past groups, I had learned to speak very precisely and in short sentences. Doing so is much less difficult on the person doing the translation and, of course, the participants learn more easily. It was hard work, but always worth the effort.

Group discussions ranged from attitudes about the visually impaired to employment potentials and possibilities for cures in the future. A large part of the discussion segment of the program dealt with how being visually impaired affects people's daily lives. No matter where they live, they have the same challenges. Transportation, shopping, and feeling in control. All over the world, these are the most common concerns of the people I have worked with. At the very deepest level is the question of self-esteem. People with disabilities commonly feel inferior to "normal" people. Our inability to function easily in a sighted world is often turned inward, causing us to feel wrong or inadequate. It's vital for everyone to realize we are not less as people because of our limited vision.

As we get to know one another better, I find laughter is the best release for stored-up negative feelings. We all have common shared experiences— hitting our heads on open cupboard doors, tripping over unexpected obstacles, bumping other people, sitting down on a chair that isn't there, putting clothes on inside-out, wiping our mouth with our jacket instead of our napkin. Sharing these incidents in a group and laughing about our clumsy attempts to be "normal" always promotes healing in our battered inner selves.

I usually start off the discussion by telling how I was once taken out to dinner and, in the dark restaurant, sat down at the wrong table. Both my friends and the complete strangers I was sitting with were in a state of shock. Fortunately, I was able to laugh at myself, which was much healthier than getting upset about it. Most participants can easily relate to those feelings.

The sense of not being normal or perfect was a special challenge in Germany, where it was much more difficult to overcome. The Germans have a long history of regarding themselves as a superior race of people—healthy, strong, and fully functional. Hitler didn't try to exterminate only Jews and Catholics. He also targeted the disabled for terror and death by gas. To this day, the attitude of many people in Germany regarding their own disabled is archaic at least and barbaric at worst. For example, a few members of our group had yellow stars on their jackets. Curious, I asked if they belonged to a club. Their answer astonished, shocked, and sickened me. I learned that they are requested by the government to wear the stars to identify them as visually impaired! Shadows of the 1930s haunt these people. I think the issue will need to be addressed if the larger population is to realize that isolating citizens with disabilities is no better than doing what was done during World War II.

And on a larger scale, leaders worldwide need to examine how their countries treat those among their populations who need and deserve special attention—the young, the old, and the physically and mentally challenged. Until a better understanding and recognition of these people's needs comes about, true civilization cannot be said to exist.

⟨❦⟩

In spite of our group's closeness, I was becoming concerned. No one seemed to be experiencing significant changes in vision. They were overly cautious, to the point of denying progress I might point out. On one hand they wanted desperately to improve, but on the other they didn't truly believe it was possible. That was not an uncommon experience for me to confront and deal with in the classes, but my German friends were a little more stubborn than most people I'd worked with.

Then, two days before the end of the class, Patricia came to the morning session with a huge grin on her face. Adolf, her new unofficial grandfather, noticed her smiling face and asked what she was so happy about. Dea was excited as she translated Patricia's response for me. Suddenly, I could barely hear them speaking, because all the participants were on their feet, hugging one another, laughing, even crying. Before Dea could finish, I realized she was reporting a major improvement in Patricia's vision. Excitement welled up in my chest and I was about to burst with pride and joy.

"Thank God," I whispered to myself. It was a joyous day. We all wanted desperately for this young girl to see better. Getting around was obviously so difficult for her; she often stumbled and ran into things and hurt herself. This change made a wonderful difference.

The last two days of our time together seemed to float by. We were all riding high because Patricia's vision had definitely improved. Her ability to walk unaided was obvious to us all. The group members were unselfishly happy for her, though they weren't yet aware of any major changes in their own eyes. I reminded them that children often show results sooner and that adults, who have older cells, may require more time. I also reminded them that these techniques had worked for many others in the past, so they had every reason to keep using them now and not lose faith.

I also always attempted to boost their expectations by informing them of current research. The most exciting potential cure is retinal implant surgery. Research is progressing in a promising way. Dr. Martin Silverman, a brain research scientist working in a small lab at the Center for the Deaf in St. Louis, Missouri, has successfully implanted healthy tissue into the retinas of laboratory animals. Early results show this procedure not only works to prevent further loss of sight, but may also even restore sight! Before long, Dr. Silverman is likely to be testing his research on humans. His work is the most promising I have come across. The possibility of a cure in our lifetime is tremendously exciting.

Closing day for our group came too quickly. It was Friday, October 13th, the time of a full moon. All the signs were pointing to an eventful day and night!

At the end of each group, we go around and talk about what we learned from the course, what we experienced, and what we all hope for the future. It is a time for reflection, for thanks, for saying goodbye to one another. It is a wonderful, spiritual experience. Usually we cry lots of tears, but more than that, we share a great deal of love. Most members usually request a group picture, a permanent record of our time together.

As we were waiting for Stephan to take our "graduation" picture, Adolf suddenly started crying and talking fast. In one of the most amazing moves I have ever witnessed, Adolf grabbed me in his arms and began to hug and kiss me. This was the man who had so obviously seen me as an enemy at the beginning. Yet here he was, overjoyed and sharing something with me! At first I thought it was gratitude for my having been able to help Patricia, his new best friend, but as it turned out, Adolf had been able to see Stephan standing in the sunlight, twelve to fifteen feet in front of the group. Adolf had not been able to see clearly or at a distance for many years! Well, the crowd went wild. Our goodbyes took hours before the last departing friend had left.

Exhausted and emotionally spent, I collapsed in a chair. Dea and Stephan were still there, and I was grateful for their company. Later we all went to dinner to celebrate the end of such a wonderful class.

⚬⚬

When we came out of the restaurant, the sky was velvet black. The moon was full. It had been a magical day and now the Universe was closing the night with a free light-show from space. Bathing in the glow of the wonderful moon, we locked arms and walked happily to Stephan's car.

Stephan asked if I'd had a chance to go to the top of the Black Forest mountain that guarded the city. I hadn't. In a burst of childlike excitement, I asked, "Can we go now?"

Within minutes, we were on our way.

We stopped at the apartment for a few items— warmer clothes and candle lamps. Dea picked up something I wasn't familiar with, called runes— small stones with cryptic marks on them that can be used for a kind of fortune telling.

Off and up toward the mountaintop we went, with Stephan determined to reach the top before midnight. Snow had been falling earlier and the drive was right out of an amusement park's rocketship roller-coaster ride. All I could see were trees the car's headlights spotlighted along the road as we wound to the top. We seemed to be drawn, up and up, higher and higher, as though we had a deadline to meet for some unexpected event. We were breathless as we reached the top.

A brisk wind had blown the snow clouds away. As I got out of the car, no one was in sight. I could not see one single artificial light. The cold wind took my breath away at first, but I bundled up and turned to look at the moon. My God! It looked so huge, so close, I felt I could reach out and touch it. My head was spinning with the awesome beauty that surrounded me.

We were all very quiet, as if we were in a church. I turned my back to the moon and stared up at the sky. Tears filled my eyes, making the view even more startling. I was overcome by an energy I had never experienced before. I was looking into space, but instead of the black curtain I usually see with my limited sight, I was given an awesome gift. I saw millions and millions of stars! Feeling mesmerized, I stared, gazing at a once-in-a-lifetime view.

I became aware of another unfamiliar sensation, as if my entire being were absorbing energy from the stars. I felt as though every single cell in my body was being charged, swelling with the midnight light source in a way reserved only for magical moments like this. I never before had such a feeling in my body. I saw millions of tiny sparkles of light, billions of miles from where I stood; and at that moment, I was able to actually feel the physical impact they have on our planet. I thought I would float off into the black velvet sky.

I just stood silently bathing in the glow of that starlight, soaking in the sense of warmth, like a cat basking in sunshine streaming in the window.

After a few moments I whispered to Stephan, who had perfect vision, to verify what I was witnessing. I began to wonder if I might be dreaming all this. Stephan stood behind me, angling his head to match mine, so he could accurately tell me what I was looking at. His voice sent chills up my spine.

"My dear Grace," he said with awe, "you are looking at the Milky Way!"

The Milky Way? I was over forty and for the first time in my life I saw the Milky Way. God is good. And, there really is a Milky Way. My heart skipped with joy at the gift I had been given in that country so far from my home.

Then, at the stroke of midnight, we sat in a circle in a clearing on top of the mountain, with the full moon shining down on us. I felt as though we were enacting an ancient ritual practiced by our forebears generations ago. Like mystics in times gone by, each of us threw the stones, the ancient fortune-telling runes, sensing deeply and instinctively that we were in tune with nature as we sat there. Everything felt right, even to the rune I drew, which displayed the symbol for "spiritual warrior." This had, indeed, been a most magical day and night.

No, I wasn't surprised that the Berlin Wall fell a few days later. Somewhere deep inside I felt that the Universe can give us the gift of seeing stars and of being one with nature, then certainly whole countries can change course midstream in the river of history. Why not?

My heart has a warm spot for the people of Germany now.

19

BACK FROM THE HIGH LIFE

After completing my course in Germany, I took a weekend to visit friends in England before going on to Spain. That's where I heard something that jarred me to the insides of my bones. San Francisco had just been jolted by a powerful earthquake!

I was in a cab, driving to London's Heathrow Airport to catch the flight to Spain, when the driver turned to me and said, "Terrible thing, eh, Luv? That earthquake in San Francisco?" For a moment, I thought he was out of touch with reality, since the only big earthquake I knew about happened in 1906!

When I finally realized he meant now, I felt sudden shock. Images of buildings falling on people and cars came rushing to my mind. I cried tears of sorrow for the pain and tears of worry for the unknown. Was my family all right? Was Ru safe? I left him on his own, since he was too old for a sitter now. He was grown up enough to take care of himself, as long as I had family and friends checking on him once in a while.

The news at Heathrow confirmed my worst fears. All airplanes to San Francisco were grounded. The damage to the airport in San Francisco was extensive and several more days might pass before planes could land. My mouth was dry. I craved information as an addict craves drugs. The phones were no help. I'd never learned to use the public phones in England. They were too complicated. In fact, the pay phones of the world are a mystery to me, which usually saves me a great deal of money. But that day, my ignorance really got in my way. It hampered my ability to find out if everyone I loved was alive and well.

My body wanted to get back to California. But my mind said go on to Spain, fulfill the contract I had made. People were waiting to see me, to work with me and the program. They were losing their sight and wanted a chance to save it, to fight as I had.

As I thought about my commitment to them, I was amazed at how small the world seemed, for the people in Spain heard about my program from satisfied graduates of a workshop I gave in Brazil, whom they met at the Moscow Eye Treatment Clinic. This network of people who knew about my work had become more extensive than I might ever have imagined. (I also worried that the KGB would get wind of the Russian Connection and come after me. Yes, I had read too many spy novels. My vivid imagination does, however, keep a little spice in my life.)

Reality was too spicy for me right now, with a major earthquake at home when I was nowhere near. People in a little city near Barcelona were depending on me and I couldn't disappoint them. They had changed their lives to attend my program. All I could do was plug in the earphone on my Walkman and tune to news stations, hoping to hear something about the aftermath of the largest quake to hit Northern California in over eighty years.

I tried to eat, but my appetite was nonexistent, my nerves screaming. I was uptight and stressed beyond words. It was time to practice my stress-management techniques. With the greatest effort, I forced myself to let go, to relax. Doing so was hard, but at least it helped a little. I had to relax, otherwise all my usable sight would fly out the window, which at that moment was about thirtythousand feet over the Mediterranean.

I was met at the Barcelona airport by my host and his secretary, who spoke English and helped me get my luggage through customs. My first words to them were about the earthquake in California and could I please use a phone?

They had heard the news, but I don't think they fully realized I was from the San Francisco area and my family might be hurt or even dead.

Communication always seems to suffer on the way from one language to another—especially if the person trying to com-municate is holding back hysteria as I was—and though the secretary spoke English, she wasn't a professional translator. My mind wasn't at ease nor was I concentrating on making small, simple sentences. I was rambling, nervous, talking at a fast, high-pitched clip. That's not the way to make a translator understand what one is trying to say. I knew better, but couldn't help myself.

Instead of being taken to a phone, I was driven to a downtown restaurant—after we went by the site of the 1992 Summer Olympics. This was turning out to be some kind of nightmare. I wanted to phone home and I was getting a sightseeing tour before lunch. Normally I would have loved taking in the local sights and getting a sense of the new country I was visiting. Not today, though.

The table was crowded with people wanting to take my course, along with mothers and fathers of children who were losing their sight. They were anxious and overly gracious all at once. My mind was spinning in hundreds of different directions. I was dizzy and had to calm down. I took some deep breaths, centered my mind, and asked the Universe for guidance and help. My priority was to be here for these people. I could feel their intensity as they tried to speak to me through a sweet but inexperienced interpreter. The messages were clear.

Could I help them? Would their children, their husbands, their wives, sons, brothers, and sisters be able to see better? Would they then be able to stop the progression of blindness, as I apparently had? These were the questions uppermost in their minds.

My inner voice wanted to scream, "Are you all crazy? Don't you know my son may be dead or buried under rubble and I don't know where he is or how he is?" I felt like a fraud at that moment. The stress was causing my vision to deteriorate. How could I tell these desperate people I might not be able to help them, since I felt totally blind at that exact moment? I wasn't, but felt like I was.

A handsome, well-dressed older gentleman named Jorge joined us for coffee and dessert. An educated man, a banker, he spoke excellent English. Realizing he understood me perfectly, I turned to him for help. Desperate, I pleaded for him to help me get to a phone so I could call home.

Jorge snapped his fingers and the owner of the restaurant was at our table in a flash. Jorge made a fast explanation. I was immediately presented with a cordless, portable phone. The owner's private phone.

I dialed home. No luck. The operator said all lines to the San Francisco area were inaccessible due to the emergency situation. How frustrating. I would have to live with this tension a bit longer. In fact, three full days would pass before I could talk to my son and discover what happened. Waiting to find out how Ru was, or if he even survived, was one of the most difficult, painful trials I'd ever endured.

One the third day, I decided to write a letter to him. Even without direct confirmation, I began to sense he was fine. The severity of the situation made me lose my inner connection and I forgot to check in with what my higher self must have known all along.

Nevertheless, the pictures on the front page of the Spanish tabloid newspaper were horrendous. Blocks of houses on fire, burning into the night. Other pictures showed buildings collapsed to heaps of rock and rubble. A horrifying picture of a hole in the Oakland Bay Bridge, with cars falling through it, made my skin crawl. The most terrifying pictures of all were of the ruined double-deck freeway, with cars and people having been trapped and flattened when the upper concrete road collapsed onto the lower one. The horror of those pictures of destruction haunted my waking moments and stayed with me in my sleep. It was making me crazy.

I was frightened, driven with worry, until I turned to a higher source for guidance. When I finally was able to do so, I sensed that Ru was fine, just fine. As a matter of fact, while writing my letter to him, I realized that if I were to choose a person to be with during a crisis or emergency, Ru would be the one. He has a way of handling things, calmly

and intuitively, and doesn't panic easily. I wrote of
my love for him and, in my heart of hearts, knew
he was safe. For the first time since the London cab
driver told me of the disaster, I was at peace.

The phone lines cleared in the evening. I
discovered that all my friends and loved ones
were well. No one had been hurt, nor had serious
damage to their property occurred. The relief I felt
allowed me to center all of my attention and energy
on the class that was just beginning.

***

The program went well. So well, in fact,
that another course was hastily put together and
I extended my stay to teach in Zaragosa, a town
in northeastern Spain. The Zaragosa class turned
out to be a wonderful experience, and nothing,
not even a bomb scare during my class, made me
regret staying on.

We met in the old part of the city, and I do
mean old (the city had a history going back 1600
years). The building was massive and housed the
International Red Cross. We met there in the late
afternoon and into the evening for the ten days of
the program.

Class started and I was working with
participants, teaching them how to work with
the pressure points, when the janitor made an
unscheduled appearance. In a tone that alerted
me immediately to possible trouble, he told us to

leave the building at once. I didn't understand Spanish too well, but I could recognize panic in any language. I didn't need the translator to interpret.

The janitor told us that a group representing the Basques called to say they planted a bomb in the building. The Basques have been fighting for separation and independence for many years, and this bomb could have been real. Fortunately, it was just a scare, but after we left the building and were safely on the sidewalk, I decided to cancel the class for the night.

My classes can get very interesting, that's for sure, and we all saw better in the dark that night, when our lives depended upon it. Motivation, as I well knew, is pretty important.

Later, instead of going to our separate sleeping quarters, we all ended up at a local bistro and laughed at our fears over a few pitchers of wine. That brought us even closer. We were survivors, with another bond to share.

❧

A young girl about seven was attending that class. Her name was Pilar and she had been diagnosed with retinitis pigmentosa. Her parents feared she would be blind before she reached womanhood. Pilar was beautiful with flashing black eyes and long, thick dark hair. She was a typical, dark Spanish beauty, who would break hearts when she was older. Somehow, she reminded me of my long-lost daughter, or how I thought my daughter might look. Not ever having seen my child after I left the hospital, I always imagined how she would look at different stages of her life. Little Pilar in Zaragosa was what I thought my child would have been like at that age.

And so I loved Pilar all the more. She became my shadow. Often, when I lectured to the class, Pilar sat beside me and held my had or touched my arm, just leaving her own hand there like a fallen rose petal, soft and wonderful. She struck a cord in me very deeply. Sometimes it troubled me and I dared not go too far into trying to understand what it all meant. Inside me were scars I didn't want to open, scars I didn't want to see.

My new friends decided to give me a going-away party, to celebrate the end of the class. There must have been forty friends and family members at the final celebration. We sat in a huge circle, and Pilar—standing proudly in the middle, so tiny, so lovely—honored me by singing a song. Her voice was pure and she sang with a maturity that was astonishing for her age.

My eyes were swimming in tears and I had to keep blinking so I could see this marvelous child. I didn't want to miss one detail. She was wearing a dress that reflected her heritage, with lace leggings and sandals with thongs that wound halfway to her knees. Her pinafore, creamy white with lace edges, covered a full dress made of wonderful designs and colors. A matching lace kerchief hugged her head, framing her sweet heart-shaped face. Beautiful, thick, dark hair cascaded over her shoulders and down the middle of her back. There wasn't a dry eye in the house after she sang. When she stopped, no one moved. Even the building seemed to miss her music, and suddenly the room itself felt lonely and empty.

I thanked God that I had been able to help these people, but especially that I had been able to be with this child. My heart was full. I had done well, staying in Spain, and all my reward was in that song still vibrating in the room.

Pilar accepted the applause and thanks, and ran to hug me. I didn't want to let her go. My heart was breaking as I said goodbye to her and her parents. Making deals with God that she would stay safe and retain her sight, I bade her farewell.

❦

Yes, we like to party, we poor-sighted people. And this, a special group, had a special party. I continued thinking about them even as I prepared for bed in my hotel room.

The knock at my door alarmed me at first. That late—it was past midnight—was not a time I was accustomed to having visitors. I went to the door, asking who it was. Immediately, I recognized Pilar's mother's voice, though I didn't understand her words, as they were in broken English, mixed with Spanish. I opened the door quickly, thinking something terrible must have happened.

Pilar jumped into my arms as the door flew open. She was crying and wouldn't let me go. After a few minutes, I understood what her mother and father were trying to tell me. They got halfway home when Pilar realized there would be no class the next day and that I was going back to California, far away. Pilar insisted they take her back to say a proper goodbye. She wouldn't stop crying until they turned the car around and headed the fifteen or so miles back to my hotel. Now we could say a true goodbye, as she knew it was going to be a long time before we would meet again, if we ever did meet again. Someday, I hope to see Pilar once more. Even if I don't, part of my heart will live in Zaragosa.

Loving little girls was very easy for me, and Pilar touched my soul. Having been deprived of loving my own child, I loved all the little girls I met. The wound in my heart was soothed by Pilar's love for me and by mine for her.

⊙⧓

When my plane landed at San Francisco International Airport on Thanksgiving Day, I almost thought I could detect the aroma of roasting turkeys in the city air. These last three months had been a special time. Change was in the air all over the world. A few days after I left Germany, the

Berlin Wall started to crumble. Chunks of the wall were being saved for posterity by treasure hunters and zealous capitalists. Ru and my friends had been unhurt by the quake. For the first time in a long while, I felt much to be thankful for on the Thanksgiving holiday.

As I waited at the airport to clear customs, not paying much attention, I unexpectedly saw someone I thought I recognized.

Walking through the automatic sliding doors to the exit area, a tall, good-looking young man with light brown hair approached me. His face was sporting a broad grin. It dawned on me that this person was mine. Ru decided to surprise me and meet me at the airport. Being home was good, but nothing felt as good as that first hug and kiss I got from my son. The world was back in its right order. Ru and I were together again, safe and sound. This was the longest time we had been apart in his whole life. And in our separation, the world turned upside down. With the earthquake and the collapse of the Berlin Wall, history had been written.

On the way home, I found out the second reason he came to the airport. He wanted to tell me the latest about his girlfriend Christy. They had been going together for almost two years and were very serious about one another. Christy had some trouble at home and, according to Ru, was kicked out of her house. Not wanting her to live on the street, he asked her to stay with us.

Since I wasn't there at the time and since no one else was around to prevent the plan from working, she and Ru... well, they were living together. The deed was done. I felt if I said she had to find another place, Ru would go with her. I wasn't ready to take that kind of a stand. I wasn't ready for my son to go out on his own. He was six weeks away from his eighteenth birthday and still in high school. He had no job skills. Also, I had a different picture of how we would end our time of living together.

Ru was my best friend, the most dear person in my life. I didn't want to risk losing him. So I made it okay for Christy to stay. But I pointed out that if they were going to play house, they must take on adult responsibilities. I asked them to make sure they were practicing birth control, as well as to pay their share of rent and household expenses. This was an effort on my part to give them a taste of adult reality. Secretly, my plan was that they would tire of being responsible and go back to being children. In no way could I protest that what they were doing wasn't right. After all, I had raised Ru for his whole life as a single parent. Having never married, who was I to preach to these young people? I felt honesty was the best approach and we began to live as a family.

Living together wasn't the cakewalk I hoped it would be. The time we spent, however, was very enlightening to me. In some ways, it was preparation for what was to come, for his finally leaving home. Of course, I knew it would happen someday, but I imagined he would first be a self-sufficient, independently successful adult. He wasn't quite there yet.

❧

For five years, my focus was international. Three or four times a year, I took two-week trips to various parts of the world, presenting seminars and working with people who had serious eye problems. But I was generating no publicity in the States, so my resources here virtually dried up. It was a difficult period all the way around.

About that time, the work I was doing internationally seemed to reach a natural conclusion, which meant things came to a general standstill. With my income significantly diminished, I could no longer afford the house. On April Fool's Day 1990, I moved in with my mother. I went from being a mother myself to being a daughter.

Even as these changes were underway, I hoped Ru would come with me, but he decided to stay with Christy and make it on his own. They moved into a friend's apartment and brought in money by slinging hash and flipping burgers.

I had been living the high life, traveling and working with people from many different countries. I experienced much success. Now all of that was in the past. My greatest regret was that my son and I weren't together. Everything else I did was a smokescreen to prevent me from feeling that loss so deeply. Spreading the pain around made it a little easier, I guess. But not much.

While putting my room in order, I kept waiting for the phone to ring. It would be Ru, asking if he could come and live with us. It never was. I still couldn't believe our life together was over. Over in one day. I was devastated and found myself crying frequently.

The pain of separation was unbearable. The empty-nest syndrome is more painful without an adult partner to share the grief. A deep depression settled into my mind, and I felt it was there to stay.

For over eighteen years I had done everything because of Ru. Even my work with retinitis pigmentosa had been motivated because of the possibility he would have it. Not only have it, but be totally blind before the age of thirteen. Originally, I accepted the eye disease in myself and only when my baby was threatened did I actively fight it. A mother's love and instinct for protection is awesome and powerful. Now, without external motivation, what would I do?

As if driven by demons, I became a model housekeeper. I wanted to do something for my mother, for her kindness in taking me in at this stage of my life. I was forty-four, and we hadn't lived together since I was sixteen. My path in life, my role, was muddied, and I couldn't get a grip on who I was anymore. This was a major identity crisis and I seemed lost in the middle of it.

❦

Unhappiness feeds on itself. Mine tripled, even quadrupled. Finally, I was able to write an article titled "Depression: Is It Me or Is It Memorex?", a silly, sarcastic fluff piece, making light of my state of mind. (It was never published.) Sitting at the computer, fingers flying over the keyboard, I wrote of all the things I was depressed about. They all came out. Looking at the manuscript on the computer screen gave me an opportunity to reflect on what was happening in my life. True, I had a great deal to be depressed about. My son hadn't even called on Mother's Day, and that just added fuel to the fire of self-pity and depression. Oh, woe is me came pouring out and it was like kerosene on a campfire. The time had definitely come to pick myself up, dust myself off, and get the hell out of Dodge.

Lost without my role as a mother and teacher, I didn't know exactly what to do with myself. After a great many hours of self-examination, I decided to write the book I had, for over fifteen years, been saying I would write.

❦

Ru and Christy were still living together. Although their housing arrangements were precarious, they were working hard to make everything turn out all right. Ru and I didn't see each other as often as I would have liked, but the times we did get together were great. He was still my best friend and I trusted him with all of my inner feelings.

He also had a sudden and unexpected confrontation with demon reality. His job as a waiter/prep cook disappeared in an overnight mystery. The owner of the restaurant where he worked pulled the plug and moved out of the building during the middle of the night, leaving no message or final paychecks for his employees. Rumors flew but no one really had the full story. All Ru knew was that he showed up the next day, on time, and had no job. It was the first major shock of his working life.

⚜

With all the changes in the world—the Berlin Wall coming down, Communism collapsing—I began toying with an idea for Ru. The way things were going for him, and given my own feeling of personal failure in not having prepared him for a successful adult life, the concept of a stint in the military sounded to me like the perfect solution. I felt confident that there wouldn't be any major wars. With the threat from the Soviet Union waning, I thought, "Who else could give the United States a problem?" With my limited understanding, I thought, "No one." I felt the lives of men and women in the military were safe enough that I could encourage my only son to join up. Weird feelings and mixed emotions intermingled with this newfound idea. After all, I demonstrated against war while Ru was floating around in the protective fluid of my womb.

He was predisposed to reject authority and war. At first mention of the words "Join the military," I imagined Ru would have an allergic reaction. I truly didn't know what he would say, but I felt it was the only way he could get more education and job skills, some-thing to prepare him for a career other than that of flipping hamburgers for minimum wage the rest of his life. It was either that or hope to win the lottery. But the experts said I had a better chance of being hit on the head by a meteor than I did of getting rich from the lot-tery. I didn't like those odds at all.

20

WAS FOUND

My daydreams were of a peacetime military—men and women working to help rebuild the nation's infrastructure, constructing low-cost housing, bridges, and roads. I felt such an experience would provide Ru with an opportunity to participate in meaningful projects.

But my initial investigations weren't promising. All the traveling we did together gave him a useful perspective on the world and the ability to function well anywhere. But it had interfered with his accumulation of school credits. He hadn't graduated from high school—though he did pass a proficiency test which allowed him to leave school and either look for employment or attend college.

Only two branches of the service accepted high school non-graduates—the Coast Guard and the Navy. But that was better than nothing. My next step was to get Ru interested in the scheme.

In the past, we'd discussed the possibility of his enlisting. It wasn't a new subject of conversation. But since Ru hadn't looked into it on his own, he was a little surprised when I told him we had an appointment with a Navy recruiter the next morning. Put off with the idea at first, he finally said, "What the heck. I don't have to sign anything if I just want to look." Off we went.

The Navy recruiter was happy to see my tall, healthy son. Ru passed the initial screening tests with flying colors, with a higher score than many of the high school graduates who applied. The recruiter was enthusiastic and offered to show us a video tape on the elite Navy SEALS. Oh boy, a movie.

We sat eagerly in front of the small television in the waiting room. It was the most exciting twenty-minute sales pitch ever developed by anyone. Navy SEALS could scuba dive, jump out of helicopters and high-flying planes, make themselves look like jungle vegetation on an empty beach, fire all known weapons, rappel down sheer mountain cliffs, and, yes, even snow ski in the Arctic!

At the end of the program, I wondered if I could join. Certainly Ru was hooked. It was remarkably similar to a camp I wanted to send him to when he was growing up, but I couldn't afford it. Here, thanks to the training of the U.S. Navy, he could learn everything I wanted him to learn. With peace breaking out all over, what could go wrong?

Ru wanted to join that day. (Never underestimate the power of television!) The bad news was that no "non-graduate" openings were available right then. However, the Navy recruiter said he would call us the moment one came up. We were both disappointed…but the Universe had something up its sleeve we hadn't expected.

Because of Ru's above-average test scores, the Navy recruiter told the Air Force recruiter, who was in the same building, about him—and Ru learned a few weeks later he could enlist in the Air Force. We hadn't even considered such an option, since the Air Force was so strict about non-graduates enlisting. How it happened, I'll never know. I think my dad, now living in the spirit world, had a hand in it. Whatever the reason, they made an exception in his case and Ru signed up. He would be sworn in a few weeks later and because he chose what was called a "deferred enlistment," he would not actually begin Basic Training for six months after that. Then he was to receive further training, as a hydraulic specialist.

I was immensely relieved, for I knew he would be taken care of physically and educationally for the next four years. My prayers had been answered. In a way, this was going to be my son's college education.

Ru subsequently took various mental and physical examinations. He came through without a hitch. His vision at eighteen was so perfect that, with a college degree, he would have been visually qualified to fly jets! That said it all for me. I felt like a million dollars. Everything might have been so different if the doctor's prediction long ago had come to pass. The years of working on Ru's vision paid off royally. Nothing could stop him now.

I knew that when he began training, the men and women in charge of the recruits would recognize his potential. There would be no limit to the opportunities he would have. Ru had turned out to be one of the most endearing, compassionate, loving young men I knew. His weak areas were self-discipline and finishing what he started. Ru was just a diamond in the rough. The Air Force would smooth out the edges, the rough surfaces, and let the sparkle show. He would shine. I felt great.

⬥

I should have known it wouldn't last.

Just a few days after Ru signed up, my blood pressure began rising dangerously. In fact, it seemed to be going out of control. For some unknown reason, it would not respond to medication. The stress-reduction program I ordinarily used wasn't working.

My doctor put me in the hospital. It wasn't just a chance to catch up on my rest, either, for my body seemed ready to blow its top. I was, he told me, a prime candidate for a stroke. His instructions were clear: stay in bed, rest.

⬥

I thought a lot about my life. I reminded myself that despite some very trying circumstances,

I felt like I had been the luckiest woman in the world—able to do the work I loved and to raise a healthy, happy son.

My encounters with people from all over the world had given me a strength I never could have imagined before. Traveling allowed me the privilege of meeting and understanding many different cultures and people. A tolerance and a love for all people in all situations gave me the courage to continue my work.

I thought of the poor farmers, two brothers, who took a class from me in Brasília, the capital of Brazil. They were uneducated and had never traveled more than twenty-five miles from their village. Yet when they heard they might improve their eyesight, they drove almost 2700 miles in a pickup truck to attend the class. I relearned about courage and determination from those brothers in Brazil.

I thought of the Hasidic Jewish father, blind in the center of his sight from early in his life, who showed me a true acceptance of everything in God's Universe. This man, one of the most loving and positive people I ever met, was a kosher chicken plucker. Kept at home because of his visual disability, he never had a formal education. Yet, while attending my course with his eight-year-old son, he was constantly being called for advice on the Talmud by rabbis and scholars from as far away as Israel. He was known far and wide for his interpretation of the Hebrew holy book and worldly scholars sought his opinion. This simple man would ask me if I minded his saying a few prayers over our fruit tree, because it was the last day to pray for fruit. During rainstorms, he gave thanks to God for watering the plants and helping the farmers. This, even if he was soaked from walking in the downpour. That gentle soul taught me humility and harmony. He never complained about his own visual difficulties. Instead, he said his duty to God was to pursue anything that might help him and his son. Humility and peace of mind were his gifts to me.

I thought of my stay with a family from the Punjab of India. Theirs was an arranged marriage; they had two children and another on the way. I lived as they did, ate what they had, and became tolerant and understanding of a way of life as foreign to me as life on the moon might be. I learned patience from my Indian sister. I had no inclination to preach women's liberation to this strong person, for whom survival was the first priority.

Her husband was my client. When I found out he had taken all their money to bring me over to work on his eyes, I returned the money to his wife. She had been furious with him, but he was the boss.

At first, I was her enemy. I was the reason food was in short supply, the reason her growing babies would not get much to eat. Yet what could she do? She was never harsh with me, just patient and kind. She taught me about sacrifice, patience, and acceptance.

I thought of my midnight journey to the top of the mountain in Germany, which taught me that magic is still in the world.

And I thought of my son, my teacher, who gave me such great lessons: unconditional love, respect for the child-spirit that dwells in us all, and the hardest one to learn—letting go.

My own life had been full—in both directions. I'd lost two children, my sight, and even a few times, my mind. Yet, there I was. Often my experiences seemed clearly to have followed a pathway that was mapped out in advance, though I, of course, didn't have a copy of the map. Sometimes the pathway rose treacherously, dangerously, as though up the side of a steep, uncharted mountain. Sometimes it led me into the presence of awesome beauty. Always it brought me to the edge, to the unknown, to discovery. By the very nature of my journey, I was always moving, seeking, yearning for a better way; I was rarely satisfied, always struggling with a certain feeling of discontent.

Except when I was working. Then all seemed right in the Universe. Being in service to others always made me feel better about who I was.

Lying in that hospital bed, I wondered what the future held for me. In spite of my general optimism, my work was at a standstill, my health was failing. To pull myself out of the pit, I was going to need help. The time had come to turn to a higher source. Had I forgotten that when life appears to be at its darkest and worst, as it did then, the greatest gift can come along?

⟨✺⟩

The phone by my bed is ringing. Not in the mood to talk, I pick it up anyway. My impatient "hello" is answered by a tiny, almost childlike girl's voice.

"Is this Grace Halloran?" the little voice asks. I'm confused. Who would be calling me here that didn't know me?

Close to being rude, I answer "Yes, I'm Grace. Who is this?"

The voice hesitates. For some inexplicable reason, everything becomes very still and quiet. The air around me feels thick and heavy. I'm aware that I'm holding my breath, anxiously waiting for her next few words. For some unknown reason, I grip the phone tighter, afraid I may lose the connection. This is an important call, although I have no idea why or who this person is. In spite of my not knowing, my entire body is on full alert.

She begins, "Does the date January 8, 1968, have any special meaning to you?" Her voice is shaky, obviously on the verge of tears.

Before I take my next breath, my mind lights up like a Christmas Tree in Rockefeller Center.

"Of course. That's the day I gave birth to my baby girl," is my instant reply. It is a date I'd never forgotten, never celebrated. It is a date etched into my memory, one that would evoke a strange mixture of feelings of joy and sorrow. The joy of giving birth, the sorrow of having left my child.

The air around me is electrified, I am straining to hear everything, almost ready to climb through the phone line to be there in person at the other end.

Instinctively, I know what she is going to say and don't dare blink for fear of missing those next few words.

"I'm that baby girl!" comes her teary voice through this mystical phone link.

Sobbing with joy and excitement, I start telling her and the world, "I knew it, I knew you'd find me! I've always prayed, always known you would find me someday!"

I am laughing and crying at the same time, just as I did those many years ago when she entered the world.

My mind is reeling. My first question pops out as though it had been waiting to leap out the moment we were reunited.

"Do you hate me?" I ask, almost afraid to hear her answer. Silently I pray for forgiveness and gentleness from her and the Universe.

"No."

Her response is a precious gift. I begin to breathe again and an overwhelming sense of well-being flows into every corner of my body and mind.

Now, with my own first question out of the way, comes the one that haunted my daughter for nearly a quarter of a century.

"Did you want me?" This is the question that made my child wonder all these years if she had been a mistake, an unwanted, throwaway, disposable baby.

She deserves to know the truth; she has suffered doubts long enough.

"Oh yes," I say. "I wanted you more than anything on this earth."

The truth. All those years fall aside, those years of thinking of her, missing her, wondering how she was. No matter what else happens, I think to myself, I can die a happy woman. My baby girl knows I wanted her. She doesn't know the circumstances, and now, if it's right, I can tell her what really happened in January 1968.

❦

My daughter lived in Santa Rosa, a hundred miles to the north. It was too late for her to drive to the hospital that night, so we made arrangements to see one another in the morning. Before hanging up, I told her she had a brother. He'd known about her all his life. I never kept it a secret from anyone in my family. They all knew my baby girl was born and that I missed her terribly. Ru knew he had a sister somewhere out there, but her learning about him came as quite a surprise.

I could hardly believe it. Ru and Christy were staying just a few blocks from where his sister lived. I called him and told him the good news. He reported to me later that the moment he hung up the phone from our conversation, he ran all the way there, all the way to meet his sister. A strange twist of fate. My son got to be with my daughter before I did. That didn't bother me. I just knew my arms ached to hold her. Sleep was a long time coming that night.

⚬❧

I was as nervous as I'd ever been in my life. Would she like me? What did she look like? Oh God, what if she didn't like me? All my fears, all my pain, kept leaping up to engulf my entire being. The last time I saw my child, I was leaving the hospital with my parole officer. It was at the hospital nursery. A window separated the two of us, just as oceans separate continents. The transparency of the glass was so misleading, causing an illusion of closeness and possibilities. My hands were pressing against the glass. It was as if I was trying to touch my baby one more time.

My beautiful baby was asleep, hands by her rosy cheeks, peacefully outstretched, totally trusting. It broke my heart to leave her there, all alone. I wondered if she slept after that day with her hands open, or had my betrayal caused her to sleep with clenched fists? Soon I would know the answer. The storm continued to rage in my soul until I heard her footsteps.

Sitting in the hospital bed, I caught a glimpse of her as she rushed around the curtain. My heart thundered in my chest. Without a word, she threw her arms around me. An overwhelming sensation of pure joy came over me. I knew now, without question, that during our long overdue embrace I had been walking around with a terrible wound. A giant wound, not only in my physical body but in my spirit as well, a wound caused by the day I left the hospital without my child.

As we held each other, rocking side to side, laughing and crying, I felt that wound finally begin to heal. My daughter's arms brought the medicine I had needed for more than twenty-three years!

Finally, as we let go, I was able to take a long look at her. She was the most beautiful young woman I had ever seen! Her beauty was much more than just physical. This was a young soul who had already paid a lot of dues in her life. But oh did her emerald green eyes sparkle! A light was shining through them. Her thick, rich, curly auburn hair framed a face that was breathtaking! This was my daughter, no mistake about it! Looking into her eyes, I could see a mirror of myself from times long past!

We began to laugh together. It sounded like crystal chimes tinkling in a warm summer breeze. We laughed and laughed, happy to be alive and together! The bonding that had been so cruelly interrupted by uncaring bureaucrats could not be broken—interrupted, yes, but never severed. She must have heard my tearful whispers when I held her in my arms moments after she was born. Those whispers had been my litany, over and over, telling her I loved her and would always miss her! She heard my voice and remembered. Because, here she was, back in my arms, and God willing, never out of reach again.

Just as I thought it couldn't get any better, my daughter brought forth another surprise. She bent down then quickly placed a soft bundle into my open arms. This was her daughter, her baby, my granddaughter! I was grateful, overwhelmed, thrilled. God was being too good to me.

The last time I held my baby girl had been in a hospital, not unlike the one I was in at that moment. Now, twenty-three years later, I was given the gift of holding my own baby's child. The circle was complete. This was a peace that only a mother can experience upon being reunited with a long-lost child. It had been a terrible and unwarranted punishment for a misdemeanor those many years ago. Holding my grandchild and my daughter, I felt peace and rightness in the Universe. I felt as if my world had tilted off its axis when I had to give up my child and had stayed off-balance for so long. Now the world was settling back into place.

The greatest possible opportunity for healing had come to me. I thought: if we wait long enough, if we keep trying to survive and help others, as I had done, then this is how the Universe says, "Thank you for being." All I know is that I am eternally grateful I lived long enough to have this chance. Instead of just surviving, I'll now be able to thrive. My daughter taught me the greatest lesson of all…

⊘≫⊘

There is a God.
And that God loves me very much!

Hundreds of years ago, John Newton, the
captain of a slave ship,
repented and became a minister in England.
He wrote a poem that has been the
hymn of millions of people. It goes,

Amazing grace! How sweet the sound
That saved a wretch like me!
I once was lost but now am found.
Was blind, but now I see.

Amazing Grace.

21

EPILOGUE

As I write this in late 1993, three years have passed since that incredible night when the voice of my daughter came softly over the phone, healing my wounded soul. Kathy—how strange it is to know her name—has now come fully into my life and I into hers. We both had deep emotional wounds, but we're healing them—together. Our relationship is rich, loving, and full of laughter. And we are working as a team to promote the eye-fitness program.

⚜

Ruchell and Christy married in January 1992. He is now completing his third year in the Air Force and his eyesight remains perfect.

⚜

I finally found out what drove my blood pressure through the roof and nearly killed me.

Doctors had discovered a small growth in my thyroid in mid-1992, but regarded it as a "normal" abnormality and gave it only scant attention. Later, though, I sought the advice of another physician, who believed the thyroid abnormality might be responsible for my dangerously high blood pressure. In May 1993, he surgically removed a benign tumor which turned out to be far larger than the ultrasound tests indicated. It had invaded my entire neck area and was putting great pressure on both carotid arteries, as well as my trachea, esophagus, and larynx.

Finding that tumor and realizing its seriousness explained a lot of things, including the general deterioration of my heath between 1986 and 1993. I was also able to make a good guess as to what caused it when I recalled my exposure to the invisible wave of radiation that spewed from Chernobyl into the planet's atmosphere in 1986.

Two months before the tumor was finally removed, I suddenly lost virtually all of my central sight. In a period of four days in early 1993, I went blind. I was plunged into despair.

I believe the enormous stress produced by the tumor was devastating to my whole being, and it went right straight to the weakest area of my body: my eyes. They were simply overwhelmed and they couldn't handle it.

Did that mean the program I worked so hard to develop somehow failed? I believe not. My purpose had initially been to prevent my son from losing his sight. At that, I succeeded. And I myself continued to have usable vision for eighteen years more than the experts predicted. Failure? In light of those achievements, I think not. My program worked, but it simply couldn't protect me against the kind of assault I experienced.

Now, with the tumor gone and my overall health on the upswing, my eyesight has begun to improve and I am again optimistic about my vision. I continue to practice my own program for enhancing visual health. Why not? It's a good program and it worked for me in the past. Furthermore, when a cure for RP turns up, I want to be prepared by having the best visual health I can. I've never given up before, and I'm not going to start now.

There is Hope for Sight!

If you have a serious eye disease, we invite you to start doing the techniques Dr. Halloran developed that can help your eyes.

The program for healing the eyes and restoring vision developed by Grace Halloran Ph.D is still going strong and is available to you today.

The Better Eye Health Program, and is run by Damon P. Miller II, MD who worked with Dr. Halloran for almost 10 years prior to her death.(1) The program has grown, but still relies on the basic principles and therapies discovered by Grace that helped her, her family and so many others regain sight. Our goal is to make this program more affordable and more available. There are tens of millions of people in this country who are losing vision due to retinal and optic nerve disease, and they need help now.

To learn more about the Better Eye Health Program, please visit www.bettereyehealth.com, where there is a wealth of information, including information about microcurrent stimulation.

To begin Grace Halloran's program, you can also contact us directly:
email: support@bettereyehealth.com
phone: (650) 948-5120, or (888) 838-3937

(1) Grace's program was the Visual Healing Program

Afterword

If you are one of the tens of millions of people in this country with degenerative eye disease, you lost a huge friend and advocate when Dr. Grace Halloran passed away in 2005. The book you just read tells the story of her fight against retinitis pigmentosa and macular degeneration, on behalf of her family and the countless others who came to her after hearing of her amazing success reversing these diseases.

However, this book does not convey the lasting importance of her work. Grace's program gives Hope for Sight to the millions still losing their sight, and will continue to restore vision to the thousands who already benefit from her program of self-treatments.

In 2001, a new program from the American Library Association (ALA) nominated 10 books about people with the ability to overcome their disabilities and these books were placed in every library in the country. The goal was to promote role models, not heroes. Grace's book, *Amazing Grace: Autobiography of a Survivor*, was in one of the first 10 chosen.

Grace persevered in helping those whose doctors insisted her therapies—and for that matter any therapies—could not reverse the course of degenerative illness. For this reason, Grace and her earliest patients are pioneers. As I write this in 2017, little has changed in the community of doctors and scientists who study degenerative illness. Today and in the 50 years since Grace first scouted the path to repairing her son's vision, most doctors continue to tell patients with macular degeneration, retinitis pigmentosa and Stargardt that they should give up hope—there is no treatment, certainly no cure.

Grace was given this sort of hopeless news herself, but her pioneering spirit refused to accept the grim news. She knew from her previous work that the body has an almost miraculous ability to heal itself. Why not the eyes? Grace believed that holistically supporting eye health could reverse degeneration and restore vision.

She was right.

Her work live on in my office and in the offices of the other practitioners she trained before she died. Most people today do a home-study program, which does not require travel. If you would like to learn more about how the *Better Eye Health Program* and Grace's work might help you regain vision, please visit us:

Damon P. Miller II, MD, CNP

- website: www.bettereyehealth.com and www.microcurrentstimulation.com
- email: support@bettereyehealth.com.
- phone: (888) 838-3937